MEDICAL DRUGS ON TRIAL? VERDICT "GUILTY!"

AN EXPOSE OF THE PRESENT DAY PRACTICE OF MEDICINE; THE DRUG INDUSTRY; AND FOOD TECHNOLOGY.

by

KEKI R. SIDHWA, N.D., D.O.

AUTHOR OF
FIT FOR ANYTHING
THE PROBLEMS OF ILL HEALTH
WORDS AND MUSIC AND ALL ALONE

NATURAL HYGIENE OF CONN.
P. O. BOX 2132
HUNTINGTON STA.
SHELTON, CT 06484

MEDICAL DRUGS ON TRIAL? VERDICT "GULITY!"

First Printing July 1976

Copyright By Natural Hygiene Press
All Rights Reserved

Printed in the United States of America

Library of Congress Card No. 76-17490

ISBN: 0-914532-13-8

NATURAL HYGIENE PRESS

A division of

The American Natural Hygiene Society

1920 Irving Park Road   Chicago, Ill. 60613

This book is dedicated by the Author
to Dr. Herbert M. Shelton,
The American Natural Hygiene Society
and to all those men and women
who have worked hard and tirelessly
to emancipate their fellow men
from fear of disease and pestilence,
and who have helped themselves, their fellow men
and the world in general
to be a little better than when they found it.

TABLE OF CONTENTS

The Message of a Sick Man to his Physician

The Message of a Sick Man
to his Physician

I want to be well
   and quietly pursue what health
   Nature gave to me;
But you stuff me with your pills,
   Leaving me half-dead,
   More ill and afraid,
Than before my cold became pneumonia.
   Can't you just for once,
   Not do something,
But be content just to be near?
   Try not to thwart nature
   Just supply all her needs;
And show you really care
   That I live or die,
   And not be a Hypocrite to your oath.

(From "Words & Music and All Alone"
        by K. R. SIDHWA)

Author's Introduction

This book has been written for one purpose and one purpose only; to put before the public, which constitutes a jury, all the evidence we can gather together in a book of this size, to enforce a verdict of "guilty" against all measures that encroach upon the life and liberty of the basic right of Mankind—health.

Henry David Thoreau once wrote:

"There are a thousand hacking at the branches of evil
to one who is striking at the root."

In the past many people have questioned the value of taking drugs when ill. At present also we are doubting, at least beginning to doubt, about whether to take the pill or not, or the outcome and future development in store when taking a trip via LSD, "pot", or heroin or the result of DDT residue and strontium 90 in our bodies. People are beginning to question, and this book has tried to put on trial not just the branches, like the question of the "pill" or LSD or DDT, which obstructs the view of the distant horizon, but the very stem and root to which these branches belong. We are putting on trial the very validity of manufacturing and giving drugs to sick people in order to restore them to health—the very foundation and cornerstone on which the medical profession solely rests its case.

In fact, when you take away a physician's drugs, powders, pills, potions, injections and what have you, he stands naked as a babe, unable to hide his ignorance on how to cope with problems of health and disease when they come before him. Deprived of his artificial armour, he is an easy prey to his own doubts and fears as to how he would "fight" disease. The whole philosophy of drug

1

medication or of Hygienic care turns on this single point, What is disease?

This book is not an attempt to convert the medical profession from its folly—nor others who are hand in glove with what Sylvester Graham called the "drugging craft" because wounded pride, professional prejudice, inordinate vanity and self-interest stand in their way of giving the matter candid and objective consideration.

In fact, we are putting them in the "witness box" to stand trial, convicted of charges brought upon them from amongst their own profession.

People of this age are rapidly losing confidence in medicine and questioning the hazards of certain drugs. In this book we are trying to give them enough data to decide for themselves to do away with all drugs and throw them in the nearest garbage can.

We want to arouse the indignation of the people to the systematic exploitation of their childlike faith. Before there can be a revolution in the care of the sick and ailing, there must be a revelation, and it is the task of any revolutionist worthy of his salt, to hasten this revelation.

In this book we have tried to take some of the commonest controversial subjects in relation to drug taking and have attempted an exposé from an Hygienic viewpoint. Many Hygienic pioneers were medical men themselves— for example, Dr. John Tilden, who practised medicine for 25 years before he saw the wisdom of throwing out all that he had stood for in the past. He was one of the numerous honorable exceptions to come out of the melting pot of medicine. As Dr. Herbert Shelton has written in his book "Natural Hygiene": "In all classes of society and in all trades and professions, the common souls compose the majority; in all these categories are to be found individual noble men to whom truth is dearer than private gain. It is the misfortune of such men in the medical society that they dare not adhere to the truth they know".

In this book we have tried to bring evidence, condemnatory evidence, against the use of drugs, from the mouths of those, who in normal parlance are supposed to be qualified, scientific, and in the know, as it were, because they have an M.D. after their name. Many have argued that medicine is scientific (it is at least experimental) and Natural Hygiene is not. The truth is just the opposite.

Medicine is not and never was a science. It is a method of treating the sick. Physiology, biology, anatomy, etc. are sciences, based on demonstrable principles, but these are not medicine. Although as a medical student you are required to study these sciences, medicine is not based on them.

However, it is indeed no small task to undertake to eradicate from the human mind the accumulated fallacies of 3000 years, to convince the people, the brain-washed public, of the fallacy of the popular idea of taking drugs for their ills, and build up a new, a different (yet old as the hills), a truer way of caring for the sick. But this we have attempted to do in this book by shocking the public out of their apathy in presenting to them what some of the enlightened medical men of the past and present era have said in relationship to drugs and their effects.

To those who would like to pursue after reading this book the principles and practice, the reasonings and applications of Natural Hygiene, there are numerous books written. In this book we have not attempted to formulate in detail the laws of life and living on which rests the materia Hygenica.

We have touched in general upon the "new concepts of health" on which the materia Hygenica rests, in the chapter of the same title. We have also tried to explain what Natural Hygiene is up against, in getting its message through to the masses and how important it is that the education of the masses is long overdue and should be tackled with all the resources available to the Natural Hygiene movement.

Some may accuse us of having spent too much time, thought, and energy in criticising medical practices instead of simply presenting "Natural Hygiene" and getting on with it. But it is necessary to expose the popular fallacies, even though old and hoary with age they may be, in our attempt to make it clear the fallacy of treatments and drugs, because the object of a "Natural Hygiene" revolution is to show people what is wrong as well as to teach them what is right.

Most of us are so conditioned by our upbringing that we made a God out of our physician and an angel out of our pharmacist. But in spite of all this, the careful and intelligent reader of this book will not miss the fact that, amidst all the sophistry and secretiveness of this divine right of drugging, the world is witnessing a breakdown of so-called medical science. The best men in the medical profession have no remedy to offer for the decline that is so obvious. People are getting fed up. Some young medical graduates are even beginning to doubt the validity of what they have learned as for example one nameless physician, when interviewed by a reporter and reported in the underground paper International Times (IT) of April 9, 1970. Our attempts are justified in that they serve to open the eyes of the people a little wider and make them see that amidst the welter of a false sense of security, the medical profession itself is not happy with the outcome.

We will feel content if in this contribution to Hygienic literature, we can awaken the average man in the street so he will not be caught in this whirlwind of medical fallacy and will open his eyes to what lies in store and to what an average and inglorious end he can come, if he continues to play ducks and drakes with his God-given vitality and flirts with one drug and another in the false hope that the gates of heaven will be opened to him. He may find the gates open all right—but from what you are about to read—you will agree that they very nearly will be the gates of HELL.

CHAPTER I

The Hue and Cry About The Pill

"You think you go to the doctor because you are ill; I think you are ill because you keep going to the Doctor."
—J. Seate.

"Sustained faith in medical 'cures' is most commonly acquired by a voluntary suspension of observation and reason."—J. Seate (Any Change is Progress).

The Pill is on its way out. In, is an "operation that gives a rest from babies", so says a headline in the London Daily Express of March 3, 1970. The article goes on to say: "The problem of mothers needing a rest from babies may be solved by an experimental operation begun by a west country Gynaecologist.

"And one of his first 'guinea pigs' is to be Mrs. Jean Seabrook of Dart Avenue, Torquay. Mrs. Seabrook, age 27, has three children, and hopes for more in a few years. In the meantime she wants to remove all fears of pregnancy. The new sterilisation technique, pioneered in Australia, makes that possible for her. It involves a simple operation lasting about 30 minutes and a four-day stay in the hospital. The ovaries are placed in a plastic bag, which isolates them from the fallopian tubes, so preventing conception.

"Later the operation can be reversed to make the woman fertile again. In Mrs. Seabrook's case that will be in at least two years. She said yesterday: 'The gynaecologist suggested this operation when I went to him for a termination of pregnancy. I just couldn't cope with more children at the moment. There must be thousands of women like me. The Pill did not agree with me, and a coil did not work' ".

The fanfare and publicity which ushered in the era of "The Pill" from 1950 onwards is now about to be forgot-

5

ten as new techniques come on the horizon. But this is the way with all so-called Wonder Drugs—they come in like lions and go out like lambs.

The population explosion stories were a preliminary buildup for the pill. Despite two world wars and many smaller ones, despite epidemics and famines, despite the "killing them to cure them" techniques of the medical profession, and despite the increased use of the means of birth control, the population of the world continues to increase.

In the past there was a fear of racial suicide, and all sorts of encouragements were given to the public to produce more babies—to be killed in war, to work in factories and mines, or just as cheap labour for the powers that be. Now we have the gadgets and the machines. Human power is not required, and another scare is thrown about—"stop multiplying yourself", with some outrageous reasons.

Not that we are in favour of unlimited multiplication, but we disagree with the false claim that the earth has reached its capacity to feed the growing population.

Way back in the 1920s Prince Kropotkin in his book "Mutual Aid" wrote that Britain could easily feed a population of 80 million people, if food was grown and husbanded along proper lines. Today we are still short of that figure by 30 million people, and yet the clarion call has been ignored. If people in Britain cannot adequately feed themselves, then the fault lies not with the growth of population, but with the methods and madness of those who are turning our soil into depleted deserts and wasteland.

But that is another chapter. In the beginning was man, and he was reproduced in the image of his forbears. And it is with reproduction that we are concerned.

Man has throughout time practised some form of birth control, and aided and abetted by nature the population problem remained constant.

However, this is an age of "instant surrender", and together with instant sex must go instant contraception. What more plausible than to find a drug that will do this?

Perhaps this era of the last 30 years or so will go down in history as an era when men ran to their bathroom cabinet to take some pep pills to wake themselves up, took sedatives to counteract their effects by mid-afternoon, and finally took a sleeping pill to put themselves to bed and start all over again; an era of "blissful forgetfulness" from one stupor (drug induced) to another, except for rude awakenings by nightmares (also drug induced) too horrible for any sanity to be preserved.

In such a drug-orientated society, where the remedy mentality prevails amongst both the lay public and the orthodox medical profession, the coming of the Contraceptive Pill was a foregone conclusion.

As soon as it was discovered and confirmed by research experiments, notably by Dr. G. Pincus and Professor J. Rock, that the use of various synthetic products derived from progesterone and testosterone and frequently combined with the use of an oestrogen could cause sterility in women by preventing the process of ovulation, the World's Press went mad.

Daily we read about how effective it was, how convenient it was, how easy it was, how utterly responsible it was, and finally, how cheap it was.

Too soon however, the women of the world awoke to find that it was not cheap, especially when human life and human health were concerned. Not only their own lives but the lives of their children, should they ever have any, were also in danger.

Another medical triumph had back-fired. But for those lulled into a false sense of security by the faulty promises of the pill pushers, it was only realised when reports of the so-called adverse effects began to appear in print.

For example, The Drug Trade News for April 25, 1966 carried a report from Sweden where "clinical cases of jaundice in women taking an oral contraceptive have been reported by two investigators".

The drug involved is Anovlar, but other reports cited Mestranol, Enavid, and Lyndiol also as possible causes of jaundice in a number of cases. In the report, K.E. Thulin, M.D. and Jerker Newmark, M.D., cite seven women, "all of whom had been taking Anovlar for periods ranging from 20 days to 6 months. These women, jaundiced upon admission to the hospital and without fever and other abnormal physical signs, gave no history of jaundice and "denied exposure to hepatitis".

Laboratory findings indicated abnormal liver function.

For example, in six cases, elevated bilirubin values and significantly raised transminase levels were found. Biopsies performed on these six cases showed histological changes (cellular or tissue changes) in the liver very similar to those seen in another drug-induced jaundice, that of chlorpromazine.

To support their claim, they cite a report in the British Medical Journal of March 5, 1966, which says "As this type of jaundice still seems to be overlooked, it is probable that a number of patients with jaundice of unknown etiology have in fact been suffering from oral-contraceptive drug jaundice."

They name as possible predisposing factors such conditions as icterus gravidarum or pruritus gravidarum, irregular menstruation, "pre-menstural tension" and migraine. These symptoms were found in the past histories of these patients, and they think that these factors should be regarded as contraindications of the use of contraceptive pills.

Although it was known in advance by the medical pundits that these pills give rise to some very undesirable side effects, the pill was allowed to be marketed. The reason is obvious as seen by statements made in an article in a Toronto, Canada newspaper, The Globe and Mail, of October 22, 1965, "A tiny ten cent pill is rapidly becoming the most successful new pharmaceutical produce of the 1960s. It has also brought a new prosperity to the corner drug store".

For those who are readers of Hygienic literature, this is not something new, as the medical profession and the chemical cartels go hand in hand when hoodwinking the public for expediency and gain. The drug industry is a profit-making industry, as we will show in our exposé, since drugs cannot touch, let alone remove, causes of disease. This is not innocent play acting; it has the sinister purpose of maintaining the highly profitable, but equally destructive, cult of the drug. A gullible public, with the shortest of memories, pays the price in ever increasing chronic disease and misery.

The enormuos profits derived from the manufacture and sale of contraceptive pills account for much of the writings that have come about the harmlessness of these drugs. We have a sinking feeling that the Pill will not be so easily forgotten and will be kept as a background contraceptive, because of the profit from it.

It is, however, safe to say that as the use of the Pill is continued, more and more so-called side effects will come to light.

From a hygienic standpoint, we cannot condone the Pill. It contains substances which suppress the normal bodily rhythms of hormone secretions. To be effective, the product must be taken regularly throughout a woman's reproductive life (like all drugs), and the method is fraught with dangers, besides being entirely contrary to the principles of natural, healthful living.

The most disturbing factor is not so much the immediately apparent adverse effects which may, or may not appear, and which may include a loss of interest in intercourse, as the long-term changes are brought about in the body's normal secretions for half a lifetime. These effects may not become fully apparent until the Pill has been in use for forty years, and if serious adverse effects should become apparent, it will be too late to do anything for those women who have used the method during that period. No one can possibly know what will be the effects of this physiological interference at the time of menopause, but they could be serious.

Also, evidence has built up that the use of this Pill (and there are 20 different kinds in Britain alone) carries with it certain visual hazards, as well as a certain liability to strokes or cerebral haemorrhage and other conditions involving blood clotting. Reports of eye troubles following their use come from the United States, Canada, and Australia.

A Montreal psychiatrist, Victorin Voyer, M.D., stated in 1966 that the pills make women more masculine and have a "deep psychological impact" upon many women. According to him "Many of them seemed to be almost in a state of unreality, like they were intoxicated, almost as if they were alcoholics".

"I am convinced it is because of the Pill. When you eliminate ovulation, you eliminate the stimulus that makes a woman feminine. It makes her less interested in being a wife and a mother".

The Lancet of June 2, 1962 said: "Twenty years may go by before we can be sure about the safety of the present oral contraceptives; and in a fortunate and well-fed country where other methods of contraception are available and effective, it seems sensible to restrict their use to those menstrual irregularities that must be corrected, or to those circumstances where other methods of contraception are impossible or ineffective".

Warnings galore have been given by the medical press as well as the lay press, but the prospects seemed so promising that the fortune-hunting drug industry refused to heed such warnings, and the marketing of "The Pill" was even boosted.

The Medical Letter of June 10, 1960 made it quite clear when it said, "no physician can feel completely confident that longterm use will prove safe for all patients". But Dr. E. A. Garrard, in his inaugural address on becoming President of the British Medical Association in 1964, spelled it out in no uncertain terms when he said, "It may be many years before we really know about their safety . . . meanwhile, it should be quite clearly understood by everyone, and I include husbands here, that if a woman takes drugs of this kind for social, rather than therapeutic reasons, they are taking part in a mass experiment—call them guinea pigs if you like . . ." The question that must be asked is "what price the convenience of the Pill"?

In order to sidetrack their customers from the dangers of the Pill, the drug companies brought out sequential forms of the Pill (C-Quens, Ortho-Novemso, Oracon, Norguen) and boosted them. Instead of taking a combination tablet on each of twenty days, a woman on a sequential regimen takes an oestrogen tablet on some of those days and an oestrogen/progestogen tablet on other days. But the risks are not less. The late Gregory Pincus, a co-discoverer of the Pill, was quoted in The New York Times Magazine of April, 1966 as saying, "I see absolutely no advantage in sequentials". Apart from carrying the same amount of risk in taking the sequentials as the combination tablet, the women face a greater hazard of having a pregnancy than with the Pill.

The reader must read this book with regard to the implications that go beyond the Pill. We wish you to question the blind unquestioning faith in technology which takes for granted the capacity to make or build something as the rightful reason to do so, at the same time believing that because we have built it, we must use it, and without doubting that such results would be inevitably beneficial. Our experiences with the atomic bomb, DDT, fuel combustion, pollution, etc., make us question such assmuptions. René Dubos, the Nobel prize winner, wrote in January 1968 in The New York Times, "Since we make so little effort to investigate the effects of social and technological innovations on human life, we are practicing— not by intention but irresponsibility—a kind of biological warfare against nature, ourselves, and especially against our descendants".

Let us look briefly at the possible effects of the Pill on the offspring and on the chance of having an offspring if one changes one's mind and decides to have it.

Dr. P. C. Steptoe reported in the British Medical Journal of March 30, 1968 on an analysis of the ovarian tissue of women who had been on the Pill for three or more years. He warned that long-term use "carries with it a definite danger of producing irreversible sterility". Later on we will show that the Pill has a sort of rebound effect also on the fertility of the individual woman taking it. To say the least—look at it anyway you like—it has an unpredictable effect and is not at all reliable as it was first made out to be.

Some findings report concern about the effect of the Pill on the genes, which are responsible for transmitting hereditary characteristics, and the chromosomes, which carry the genes. Dr. John A. McCluskie of Celebe, New South Wales, in a letter he wrote in the May 13, 1967 issue of the Medical Journal of Australia, said: "The indiscriminate use of hormones may well rank worse in mutagenic (gene changing) developments than will those in the indiscriminate use of X-rays and radioactive fallouts".

Another physician, Dr. David H. Carr of McMaster University in Hamilton, Ontario, said: "Chromosome abnormalities were found in six of eight abortuses (aborted fetuses) collected from women who became pregnant after using oral contrapectpives. . . ." as reported in The Lancet of October 14, 1967.

On April 26, 1968, The Medical World News quoted Dr. Cecil B. Jacobson as saying, "Damage sown in the germ plasm is far more dangerous to the human race than immediate clinical complications like cancer or thalidomide, which cripple or kill a single person but are not reproduced".

That the taking of the Pill has far-reaching effects no one doubts, and every day new discoveries are taking place as to the influence of this menace on society. Since November, 1966 the Food and Drug Administration, acting on a recommendation by its advisory committee, has called for uniform labelling on all pills sold. The uniform labelling says: "A small fraction of the hormonal agents in oral contraceptives has been identified in the milk of mothers receiving these drugs. The long-range effect on the nursing infant cannot be determined at this time."

Also, according to the British Medical Journal for September 9, 1967, and the Obstetrical and Gynaecological News for December 15, 1968, it has been established that a decrease in the milk supply occurs in a significant share of mothers on the Pill.

Also, the giving of the Pill to teenagers is reported as giving a great deal of concern to many physicians who feel that the pituitary gland may be affected and also "That use of these compounds may lead to premature closing of the epiphyses (the centres near the end of the long bones), with consequent retardation of growth of the bones."

But this is what is to be expected. You cannot meddle with life's functions without getting hurt in the process. The idea that we can solve the world's economic, moral, or any other problems by giving pills to women is as ridiculous as putting an ambulance down the valley instead of providing a fence on the cliff top.

Almost from their introduction, the birth control pills have been implicated in diseases involving blood clotting. The Philadelphia Inquirer for April 29, 1966 carried a report by David B. Clark, M.D., professor of neurology at the University of Kentucky, saying that the incidence of vascular problems in young women has increased significantly with the use of birth control drugs. He made this remark when he discussed a paper by a team of neurologists from the University of Miami, which outlined cases of severe headaches, epileptic seizures, and cerebral oc-

clusive incidents (haemorrhages) in women taking contraceptive pills.

The use of contraceptive pills also causes enlargement
of the breasts as well as other tissues of the body, due to
water retention. To many of the women this does not
seem sinister, but from a hygienic point of view it means
a failure of elimination, which could contribute to a
"dropsical" or uremic condition. Water retention entails
considerable and widespread weakening of tissue strength
and function throughout the body.

That is one reason why many women on the Pill put on
weight. Tablets whose progestogen is one of the hortestos-
terone derivatives are more likely to add tissue protein—
which is firmer and more difficult to dispel. The taking of
any drug puts a great deal of distress on the liver and the
kidneys, two important eliminating organs of the body.
Hence, hepatitis and nephritis are common side-effects of
the Pill.

Other "side-effects", so called, and remember, they are
all pathological, are nausea, irritability, cramps, weariness,
and vaginal discharge. Periods will usually get scantier,
though they may become heavier.

Disturbances of sleep, general nervousness, drying of
the vagina, and trouble with varicose veins are also known
to occur. Also, in some women ulceration of the corneal
window of the eye is liable to occur.

In one study of the Pill, the body's metabolism of
glucose (as indicated by the glucose tolerance test) was
altered in 27 percent of those with a family history of
diabetes, and in 18 percent of those without such a history.
Together with other laboratory evidence, this has raised
suspicion that the Pill might precipitate diabetes.

It is also admitted that the Pill may aggravate certain
ailments—e.g. asthma, eczema, vasomotor rhinitis, and
migraine. Some women's varicose veins do become a little
more prominent on the Pill. The same goes for broken
veins.

It has also been admitted that people suffering from
the following symptoms and diseases should stay away
from the Pill; otherwise, the disorders are liable to worsen:

They include liver disease like jaundice, thrombo-
embolism of the lung, or thrombosis in a deep vein.
Other symptoms where the Pill is contraindicated are

in diseases of the pituitary gland, in cases where there is undiagnosed bleeding from the vagina, cancer of the breast and uterus, diabetes, severe mental depression, heart disease, and epilepsy. Other side effects of taking the Pill are visual defects, e.g. sudden, partial or complete loss of vision, double vision, protrusion of the eyes or sudden migraine.

Fibroids already present sometimes enlarge when a woman starts taking the Pill. Thinning of the hair over the temples and forehead is a common experience and patchy loss of scalp hair (alopecia areata) has been reported in women taking the Pill—so have backache and itching.

Even the skin on the face appears to go brownish in patches. Hyperpigmentation thus occurs. Sometimes sunlight dermatitis may occur in a woman taking the Pill.

You name it, my friends, and the Pill has got it in for you. Even cancer of the breast and uterus are suspect, and there was higher than average occurrence of congenital abnormalities in babies in cases where the mother was given medicinal treatment with large doses of progestogens in the first thirteen weeks of pregnancy.

The irony of it all is that it has been found that the taking of the Pill makes some fertile women unusually fertile after stopping the Pill. Sixtysix percent in the first month (U.S.A. trials) and 80 percent in the first two months (U.K. trials) conceived rapidly after stopping the Pill.

The Sunday Mirror (London) of March 8, 1970 carries Back Page headline "Pill Firm Sued Over Wife's Death".

The Pill concerned was Volidan 21, used by Mrs. Eileen Davies, a 28-year-old housewife of less than a year. Volidan 21 was one of the eleven pills cleared in December (of 1969) by the Government's drug safety committee. Mrs. Davies died in January 1969 due to pulmonary embolism—a lung obstruction caused by thrombosis. Her husband, Peter Davies, is suing the firm, B.D.H. Pharmaceuticals, a part of the Glaxo group.

Yes—Mr. Davies is right, alleging negligence and breach of duty. It is also reported that another man, a Mr. Freeman, is going to do the same because his wife also suffered after taking the Pill. If every man, woman, and child will claim compensation for the death of their relatives, the drug firms would soon be out of business. That is why we want to educate the public to abandon the use of drugs—for their own safety and for the safety of their children.

The tragedy of Thalidomide has not yet taught a lesson either to the medical profession or to the chemical cartels. How many more Thalidomide-like tragedies do we need to make the public sit up and take notice, and not put their faith so easily and so carelessly into the hands of those who only know how to prescribe a drug to suppress a symptom?

The lesson is with drugs of which we can never be sure. The whole idea of giving drugs to recover health or maintain health is brought over to this day and age from the day when witchcraft and shamanism flourished in past ages.

We hope to show in the following pages that drugs and drug-taking is the grand self-delusion of our age. Karl Marx once said, "Religion is the greatest drug." Today it is true to say, "Drugs have become the greatest religion." And the reason for this uncritical acceptance of drugs is that, in offering a seemingly easy way out of our health troubles, they appear to fulfill a requirement of perverted psychology. Man tries to "get away with it" if he can.

Meanwhile the debate continues about the advantages and disadvantages of the present oral contraceptive pill. For example, Hilde O'Hara wrote from Cornwall to the New Statesman of June 17, 1966: "Many of our clinic patients whom we thought happily settled on the Pill have changed to our more recent IUCD method, and still more would do so if only it were 100 percent effective, as is claimed for the Pill. Inquiries as to why they wish to change bring floods of confidences, e.g. 'What is the use of a perfectly safe contraceptive if you lose interest in sex?' . . . 'I just feel different' . . . 'I feel apathetic about the whole thing'. More disturbing are the women who notice no differences themselves, but whose husbands ask, 'Have you stopped loving me?', or who suffer such a drying of the vaginal tissues that they have to use a lubricant. While no ordinary man can expect the privileges of a sheik with a very large harem—a female in heat always available—he surely deserves a better fate than intercourse with a permanently pregnant (physiologically speaking) wife."

And the London Daily Telegraph of March 12, 1970 had the headline, "Warning on Heart Risk from Pill". It went on: "The birth control pill may remove women's natural protection against heart attacks, Dr. Alastair Breckenridge, consultant physician, Hammersmith Hospital, said today. 'At the moment women seem to be protected by their sex hormones. But the Pill could change that. It might cause changes in the body which put a person in a greater risk of heart attacks, raising the blood pressure, and changing the level of blood fat'.

Dr. Breckenridge continued: 'It may be that in twenty years time we shall be dealing with a population of women who, because they have changed their hormone balance at will, have the same bad outlook for high blood pressure as men'. He was speaking at a conference held by the Chest and Heart Association in London. 'At present women suffer less from heart attacks and strokes than men, and their expectation of life is four or five years greater'."

Alas, there are none so blind as those who will not see.

Dr. R. S. Morton, a British authority on venereal diseases, is quoted as saying, "The Pill does more harm than thalidomide." He is a World Health Organization consultant, and in his book *Social Freedom in Venereal Disease* he states: "The accumulation of cases of long term individual misery and venereal disease as a direct result of its use is more calamitous than anything precipitated by thalidomide."

Dr. Morton says that the Pill has made for serious moral laxity. "For the single the Pill might be classified with the most dangerous of the polluting pesticides, and was stamped with the same criteria of failure: shortsightedness, inability to foresee latent side-effects, lack of adequate field trials, too little thought and too much enthusiasm."

We read in the Life Natural of March 1973, "Gynaecologists in England, Australia and the U.S.A. have just confirmed another side-effect—the Pill can make women infertile long after they have stopped taking it."

The Lancet (London, 12 July 1968) warned of increasing evidence that the use of the contraceptive pill is linked with thrombosis. The journal Mother India (Bombay, March 1970) quoted Dr. Hugh J. Davis of John Hopkins University, U.S.A., as saying, "Breast cancers have been induced in at least five different species of animals by treatment with the same synthetic hormones being marketed in the oral contraceptives. Every important agent which has a carconogenic (cancer-causing) effect in humans has been shown to cause cancer in animals. There is no reason to presume that the single exception will turn out to be the oral contraceptives."

The medical reporter of The Times, London, wrote on 27 October 1972: "Some doubt on the finding of the Committee on Safety of Medicines yesterday that the contraceptive pill will not, on the evidence of extensive experiments with animals, cause cancer, is expressed in a leading article in the British Medical Journal.

" It says many people who feel oppressed by the increasing threat of world over-population would desperately like the Pill to be found safe from the point of view of cancer. But the Committee's studies neither incriminated nor exonerated oral contraceptives as carcinogenic.

" The Journal compares the response of the Committee with that of the Food and Drug Administration in America, which had banned D.D.T. because of an increased risk of liver tumours in mice. In the oral contraceptive studies male rats showed a pronounced, dose-relafed increased risk of developing liver tumours in response to norethynodrel alone, or together with mestranol, megestrol acetate in combination with ethinloestradiol or this substance alone, increased the incidence of liver tumours in male and female rats.

" In spite of these findings the Journal says the Committee on Safety of Medicine stated boldly that its tests did not support previous work on liver damage. Although that was strictly true, because no liver damage was encountered, the Committee's statement, the Journal says, 'sweeps a lot of liver tumours under the carpet'."

All we would tell our readers is: If and when you come across a statement in the press that the Pill will not cause cancer or . . . (some other disease) . . . please bear in mind the remarks of the British Medical Journal. IT MAY SWEEP A LOT OF . . . UNDER THE CARPET!!!

In the National Enquirer of 26th August 1973 and published in America we read of yet another type of trouble brewing when people resort to the Pill. The headlines scream at you: "Women with Contact Lenses Face Problems if They Are on the Pill." The article continues, "Women who wear contact lenses and take birth control pills may experience eye irritation and discomfort, a group of British researchers say. Anthony Sabell, of Aston University in Birmingham, England, who headed the research team, said the female hormones present in the Pill cause the eye to produce less tear liquid. Since a contact lens normally floats on a film of tears,' the lens can cause considerable discomfort if the tear film is insufficient, he said. Some opticians suggest that as many as thirtyfive percent of women experience trouble with contact lenses after taking the Pill."

Finally, to conclude this chapter I can do no better than quote to you an article which appeared in Ladies Home Journal of August 1973, published in America, in which the now famous Ralph Nader gives his report on the dangers of the "morning-after pill", a new drug which is being thrust on the beguiled public and as an improvement and an excuse for "The Pill".

Rightly Nader has condemned this in his report and a more serious indictment than this is not easily found. From this and other reports we can only hope that the Pill will eventually fade out as the people realize the dangers facing them. Following then is the full verbatim report from Ralph Nader, as published in the magazine mentioned above:—

" *There is much controversy about the 'morning-after pill,' a large dose of the synthetic female hormone DES, which is known to cause cancer in animals. Should women take this drug?*

" Many doctors are prescribing a new drug to prevent pregnancy, the 'morning-after pill.' Should you be concerned about this new form of birth control? Should you take it?

" First, you should be very concerned. The 'morning-after pill' is actually a massive does of DES, a synthetic female hormone (oestrogen) long known to cause cancer in animals and recently banned as a food additive in beef cattle. More recently, DES has been linked to cancer in human beings. In April 1971, Dr. Arthur Herbst, a Boston physician, reported in the New England Journal that seven young women developed vaginal or cervical cancer as a result of ingestion of DES B by their mothers, who took it while they were pregnant. There are now well over 100 such cases reported. These mothers were among tens of thousands of women who were given DES during the 1940s and 1950s, usually over a period of three months in early pregnancy, because doctors then believed the drug could prevent miscarriage. Belatedly DES was found ineffective for that purpose and in 1971 the Food and Drug Administration warned doctors not to give it to pregnant women.

" Now DES is becoming increasingly popular as a 'morning-after pill'. Doctors have found that when taken within 72 hours after intercourse, in doese of 25 milligrams twice a day for five days, DES is highly effective in preventing pregnancy. 'Most' university health services prescribe it, according to an official in the Centre for Population Research of the National Institutes of Health. And sales of the drug have significantly increased over the past few years.

" Researchers report that the effectiveness of the 'morning-after pill' may be as high as 95 percent. One of them, Dr. John Morris, reported in the American Journal of Obstetrics and Gynaecology in January, 1973, that of 9,000 women given the pill after intercourse only twentynine became pregnant. (This failure rate is actually higher than it may seem, since by estimate only 360 of these women would have become pregnant anyway).

" The effectiveness of the 'morning-after pill' also depends, of course, on whether a woman takes the correct dosage. Because the pill can cause violent nausea, a woman so affected might stop the medication before taking the full course, in which case she might become pregnant.

" Is the pill safe? Doctors who prescribe it generally say that it has not been proved *unsafe*. They note that as a 'morning-after pill' DES is given for a short period of time and in relatively small doses. (A daily dose of the Pill is 50 milligrams, about 500 times the amount of oestrogen the body produces in a day.) However, the Herbst report indicates that even this dosage can be dangerous to a female child if the woman does become pregnant. In one case of cancer in the daughter of a woman who took DES to prevent miscarriage, the mother had only taken the drug for ten days. In another, the mother had taken amounts of only 1.5 milligrams per day. The 'morning-after pill,' then, is not safe if a woman finds that she is pregnant after taking it.

" There is no data to show that the 'morning-after pill' causes cancer in the woman who takes it. On the other hand, as Dr. Herbst notes, 'We do not have enough data or knowledge at the present time to say what the smallest dose or the shortest duration of exposure to this drug is that could cause trouble.' If DES causes a more common type of cancer such as breast cancer (vaginal cancer in young women is very unusual), it is unlikely that conclusive human evidence will ever be available. Certain conditions enhance the chances of cancer developing: for example, if your family has a history of breast or genital cancer, exposure to DES would increase an already indicated risk and you should probably not take the 'morning-after pill.' Further, it is known that exposure to oestrogen in birth-control pills over a period of time can cause serious side-effects in some women. Thus the additional exposure from the 'morning-after pill' (which roughly equals ten months of birth-control pills) can increase the risk of cancer and other side-effects for women who have already had considerable exposure to oestrogen in other forms.

" Lack of hard data to prove that the 'morning-after pill' is safe caused an FDA advisory committee a few years ago to recommend against approving it. Last May, the advisory committee reversed itself and the FDA has now approved the pill 'as an emergency treatment only.' The FDA has notified physicians that they should give patients a pregnancy test before prescribing the pill, and warned that any woman who is pregnant or whose family has a history of breast or genital cancer should not take DES. The FDA also said abortion should be seriously considered if pregnancy does occur after taking the pill.

" You should not take the 'morning-after pill' unless these safeguards are strictly invoked and unless your doctor is willing to sit down and discuss with you the risks in your particular case. Unfortunately, many doctors have not been willing to do this. The Public Citizen's Health Research Group, a consumer organization in

Washington, D.C., affiliated with me, finds that precautions have been uneven at best, and in some cases entirely ignored. One woman in Washington, D.C., was able to get a prescription over the phone with no questions asked. Surveys by student groups have turned up equally irresponsible practices among some doctors dispensing the drug through campus health services.

" Advocates for Medical Information, an Ann Arbor group, reported last year that the health service at the University of Michigan was taking almost no precautions. A survey of 69 women who were given the pill, most of them by the University health service, found that only five women were warned about a cancer hazard if they did have a child; none were informed of a suspected cancer hazard to themselves. Only four women were given pregnancy tests; only three were asked about their family medical histories; only ten were questioned about exposure to other oestrogens; and only nine were followed up for side-effects or pregnancy. (The University of Michigan health service has since agreed to give women a fact sheet outlining the hazards of the pill.)

"ᴸ At the University of Vermont, according to a student investigation, doctors had not been checking medical or family histories for evidence of increased risk. There was no follow-up in case of pregnancy, and women were not told of the evidence of risk to the foetus or to themselves. This is typical of most universities.

" Some health services are more responsive. The Indiana University health service has prepared a written consent sheet—unfortunately used only at the doctors' option— which states that because of a strong possibility of cancer in offspring, 'it is probably unwise to continue pregnancy' if DES is not effective. The form also states that the long-term and some of the short-term effects of the pill are not known, and that the use of well-studied methods of birth control is preferable.

" These surveys were taken while the pill was still under investigation, *before* it was approved by the FDA, and while it merited the closest vigilance from doctors. The strong possiblity is that if doctors failed to use precautions when the pill was unapproved, they will be even less inclined to do so now—unless women themselves demand it.

" Here is what you can do to protect yourself:

1. Find out whether the 'morning-after pill' is available in your community. Check with campus health services, medical clinics, and your local medical association.

2. If it is being prescribed, determine what precautionary measures are taken, if any, and how they are enforced. (If doctors are given the option of handing out a fact sheet, are they actually doing it?)

3. Are doctors giving women *full* information about the pill? Dr. Sidney Wolfe of the Health Research Group recommends that before a prescription for the 'morning-after pill' is ordered each patient should be given a fact sheet to inform her that:

• DES has not proven 100 percent effective in preventing pregnancy.

• DES has been found to cause cancer in the female children of some women who have taken it.

• Your doctor should determine as nearly as possible whether you are already pregnant (*prior* to the intercourse for which the pill would be taken).

• If you have ever had breast or genital cancer, you should not take this drug.

• If there is a history of breast or genital cancer in your family, the risk to you is increased.

• Your risk is probably higher if you have been exposed to other oestrogens, such as birth-control pills.

• DES should not be used as a routine form of birth control. If you have taken it once, do not take it again.

4. Follow-up of each patient taking DES should be mandatory, and the option of an abortion offered if a woman does become pregnant.

" Women who consider the risks too great for any of these reasons may prefer to wait and see whether they are pregnant and then consider an abortion. The crucial point is that women should be informed of the facts and risks so that they can become part of the decision-making process on what affects them. "

Finally in 1976 reports emerged that two makes of contraceptive pills were responsible for causing cancer in animal tests and have now been banned. The hue and cry over the Pill still goes on and as time goes by more side effects are bound to emerge.

* * *

CHAPTER II

Drugs and Our Youth

Good-bye health, exceuse me, I
   haven't time.
Please come back, or try and wait
   just now I haven't time.
I must not sleep or rest—I
   haven't time.
I'd love to exercise, but I
   haven't time.
I can't help eating whatever's there
   For it means saving time.
I can't think, I can't read,
   I'm swamped, I haven't time.
When I am dead, you'll be gone.
   I wonder will I ever have time.

   (From "Words and Music and All Alone" by K. R.
Sidhwa)

An article by Henry Miller entitled "Drug Peril Hits
Home in U.S.", which appeared in the Daily Telegraph of
February 25, 1970 goes to show how serious the problem
of drug addiction is becoming. The opening paragraph of
this article says: "Millions of American parents have been
painfully awakened in recent weeks to a menace that
has been stalking their children for considerably longer
than many of them dare to suspect—drug addiction. All
at once, even in the best regulated homes, anxious glances
are being directed at youngsters who may have been se-
cretly snared into serious drug uses or, at the very least,
tempted to try smoking marijuana". It continues, "The
comfortable illusion that the problem of drug abuse be-
longed only in the ghetto, among the hippies or disordered
groups on the fringes of 'decent society', has been brutally

destroyed for many thousands of well-placed families. Its pervasiveness is now so great that it is striking at the homes of some of the most eminent and influential people in the land."

But should we wonder why this is happening—should we not ask, "Who makes the Dope addicts?" We believe that when we answer the above question truthfully, only then can we achieve a real solution.

Without any hesitation and unequivocally, we lay the blame for this problem on (1) the medical profession, (2) the Food and Drink industry, as we shall see, (3) the drug and chemical cartels who manufacture these poisons, and (4) on society as a whole, which has condoned such practices.

That we are not the only ones who think so is confirmed by the following article which appeared in the London Observer and was subsequently published by the Los Angeles Times of September 5, 1967 under the heading, "Briton Cites Deepening Adult Addiction":

" While young 'pot' smokers and amphetamine takers are filling headlines, adults are calmly sinking deeper and deeper into their own addiction. Dr. M. M. Glatt, who treats addicts at St. Bernards Hospital, Southall, Middlesex, warns that barbiturate abuse and addiction are being overlooked. 'Among the middle-aged', he says in the British Medical Journal, 'large numbers are either overusing sleeping pills or are already addicted to them'. He continues, 'Barbiturates are prescribed in enormous quantities, increasing year by year from 15 million in 1961 to 17 million in 1965.

'This problem among the middle-aged is second only to Alcoholism', he says. 'Deaths from barbiturates by suicide have risen from 575 in 1956 to 1,490 in 1965, and deaths from these drugs by accident have risen in those years from 140 to 525. Middle-aged women, mostly housewives with no respite from the "stress of boredom", are the main victims. They cannot escape to a pub, and instead ask their doctors for sleeping pills. Just as alcohol releases inhibitions, so sleeping pills dispel worries and induce a pleasant, hazy state. The danger lies in overuse, when they can lead to chronic intoxication, unsteadiness, and slurred speech. The withdrawal symptoms can be very

unpleasant, and in some respects, resemble those of alcoholism, with hallucinations and convulsions.
" 'Doctors have been warned repeatedly of the dangers of over-prescribing these drugs, but a rising number of prescriptions and addicts indicates that the warnings are being ignored by many doctors'."

There is nothing wrong with the young, nor with middle-aged housewives. The trouble is with our boasted civilization so that, beneath the veneer, life in the big cities is both anti-human and anti-social.

As we have said before and will say again, addiction to drugs starts from a very young age, and in some cases even before children are born. Children of those mothers who are habituated to take drugs and especially during pregnancy, have not only a chance of being born abnormal and malformed, but can inherit the addiction to these very drugs. Tranquillizers, headache remedies, bromides and other sedatives, barbiturates, are all culprits.

According to the Manchester Guardian of October 27, 1967, "The cortisone drugs have a wide application and have been used for many years. It has already been estimated in America that women given the drugs while pregnant have a one-in-ten chance of producing an abnormal child."

Some 32 years ago in 1944 an article in the American Weekly entitled "No longer any excuse for becoming a dope slave" said the same thing about being addicted to morphine. "The use of morphine to relieve suffering patients has started thousands of them on the road to drug addiction . . . Every respectable physician hesitates long and thoughtfully before he prescribes morphine for a patient, no matter how great the suffering. The doctor knows that if he has to administer the drug for a month, in sizeable doses, he has a potential morphine addict on his hands."

All these drugs are obtained only under medical supervision and prescription—the people cannot be blamed. The onus lies squarely on the physicians and the medical profession who teach people to use drugs in one way or another. The family medicine chest in the bathroom is the number one culprit to make us morons and drug-addicts.

The idea that drug-addiction can be remedied by drugs should have died long ago. Drug after drug has been employed to cure drug addiction, and while this method of treatment has often resulted in another addiction, it does not remedy the original drug addiction. Whether the drug is alcohol, tobacco, coffee, opium, heroin, or any other poison, addiction to one drug is not cured by another drug.

The St. Petersburg Times for November 1, 1967 carried a story of an experiment in Toronto, Canada, which proves our point. Leary and other advocates of L.S.D. poisoning have often claimed that this hallucinatory drug successfully combats alcoholism. But after 18 months of study, four Toronto physicians have pronounced as useless the effects of L.S.D. on alcoholism.

Drug addiction, in our opinion, also starts when people get habituated to stimulants in their diets. At present we know of a girl of nineteen who, if she is not careful, will become habituated to using stronger drugs. Her sister is already a drug addict, and the mother is hooked on tranquillizers. This girl is very fond of coffee and says she must have it; otherwise she feels awful. When she cannot get a cup of her favourite poison she takes caffeine tablets, which she carried for just such occasions. Drugs present in our diet make us habituated to their use. Chocolate and sweet eating is just one such form of stimulation. All types of soft drinks with the presence of caffeine are another. Ice cream nowadays also contains drugs and chemicals. Thus the habit starts when young, and we are hooked to the "Stimulant Delusion"; soon the same children on becoming adults seek for stronger and stronger "stimulants". The innumerable cups of tea, coffee, coca cola, soda pop, ice cream, candy, and chewing gum are left behind, or together with them they pass on to wines, spirits, beers, and alcohol of all kinds, tobacco in cigarettes or pipes, then to marijuana or hashish, opium, heroin, L.S.D., gum sniffing, methylated spirit, shoe polish, and even morphine. The habit grows, starting with a little, then bit by bit until it has finally become a habit.

Beginning in 1950 the world has witnessed what the pharmacologists refer to as a pharmaceutical "explosion". By this they mean that a great increase in the production of new drugs has taken place. During the past decade or so, some 5000 new drugs have been introduced, and new drugs are pouring off the production line at the rate of

400 a year. As every drug is a poison, every new drug means a new disease and the chances of being hooked on either one or the other drug.

Finally we would like to warn the Youth of the World that unless they themselves revolt against such practices, which by and large are condoned by society as a whole, they will have no future to think of.

Hygienic revolt is an alternative revolt. It is a path through the woods to the clearing. This path to man's highest development is choked by a variety of fears, the father of which is fear of change—change in thinking, change in feeling, change in action.

America and Europe have grown old and rich; and age and wealth are afraid of change. They resist it with all the machinery of their business institutions, their political pressures, and their massive communications media. They not only barricade themselves, but you too, behind these subterfuges, as a defence against the winds of change. This should worry the younger generation more than anything—more than communism, more than the Bomb—for this kind of stubbornness and fear is the prelude to spiritual death which precedes physical death. It is the hardening of the arteries of society, which marks its withering.

This conservatism is the real threat to your future. In its extreme forms, conservatism is an attempted return to the past. In its more moderate sense, it is the preservation of status quo. Sickness is a Big Business—the industry that is the cause of sickness and the industry that is the effect of sickness play into each other's hands. You, its victim, are indeed the SUCKER.

The major object of your vigilance now is to perceive how the government of money—far more powerful and persuasive than government of laws and justice—impinges on every sector of your life, affecting not only what you do but how you think and feel. And because it is clothed in the palpable benevolence of prosperity, you accept this impingement, if indeed you are aware of it, as normal and necessary, whether it is the commercials on television, the billboards on highways, or the trash sold to you in so-called "health literature". If you think about these at all, you consider them a small price to pay for the strictly private happiness you are free to pursue.

Perhas you will not think the price quite so small as you read these pages. If you agree that this price is getting a bit too high, then you, the young consumer citizen, will, let us hope, begin to question the structure that makes it so and the pagan prayer—Give us this day our daily profit—that perpetuates it. Not only health, but the welfare of mankind is at stake; our art, our culture, our ethics, nay, even the not-so-new science, as indeed the whole integrity of man.

The impingement of secondary purpose on primary experience is becoming far too common. Even the so-called "scientific journals" are written with the profit motive— how much will it bring?—the shadow that dogs the substance in all phases of our activity. The "Scientific journals" play up the theme that is bound to attract dollars and cents rather than factual truths, e.g. fluoridation, chemical additives in our food, and the effects of hallucinatory drugs like L.S.D. Many of you, instead of realizing that you are being sold something, simply put on your consumer's hat and accept the fact that commerce rules, and that, since the production of goods (however worthless) is the cornerstone of a nation's economy, the consumption of goods is that nation's duty. The dire result is that the sales of coffee, tobacco, cigarettes, booze, candy, tinned and packeted foodless food, cocoa, and pepsi-colas soar to an all-time high, bringing in their wake decayed teeth, hardened arteries, ulcers, cancers, and a shattered nervous system.

Selling soap powders and groceries is one thing. What riles us is the fact that the fruits of the human mind and spirit become products—in that art, poetry, writing, and the press are used to induce us suckers to buy their worthless products.

The measure of the worth of a product like soap powder is both quantitative and qualitative, but the measure of the worth of a creative act is qualitative only, and to apply the standard of one to the other is to deprive a man, whether he is an artist or not, of his reason for being.

You may argue that we are now so used to this commercial dictation in our lives that we have come to accept it as a necessary corollary to the prosperity of our profit system. You are told that it is the realistic price we have to pay for such benefits as a free press, television, and a free society.

How that word "free" is abused! Indeed, this free society is not free to discuss even partial alternatives to the profit system. As for the free press and free television, it is surely too much to expect that with their total dependence on advertising revenue, they would be free to examine impartially anything that might diminish this revenue.

The citizen has become the consumer, the individual the instrument, not of a super state, but of the super commercial market.

And is this kind of brain washing—for that is what it is—palatable to you? To me it presents some real danger. It conditions us in less obvious but possibly more harmful (in the long run) ways than that of straight-forward state control. Nobody has yet begun to gauge the effect on the mind and spirit of man of the profusion of advertisements to which he is exposed every day of his life.

Some of you will say: "But what has this got to do with this book and the question of Drug addiction? The answer is "A great deal". This book is written to tell the world at large and especially the young ones, the truth about the corrupting influence of taking drugs in any form. We are not questioning your right to take any drugs if you so wish, but we wonder if you are naive enough to believe that a change will not be effected in you if your persist in this habit of drug taking.

It is not a question of freedom or prohibition, for after all you can jump from the top of the Empire State Building, but whether you are sane enough to realize what the effects will be. It is not a question of whether you should be allowed to experiment with "pot", hashish, etc., but whether you realize that the more these habits are condoned, the greater will be the market for large-scale production—a question of supply and demand, and hence also, of profit to those who will market it, so that you may experiment to your heart's content. Whether you are aware that a sham battle is being staged, by those with vested interests, against the use of these drugs, so that a thing denied is more precious than ever, and you will want to hook yourself on to it just for curiosity's sake—a psychological bait if ever there was one.

This book shows an alternative to drug taking. This alternative is Natural Hygiene. It is a philosophy of life and living geared to the optimum benefit of the welfare of man, whereas the things we have been writing about are geared to the welfare, not of man as a whole, but of an individual or a group of individuals whose immediate motive is the welfare of their bank accounts. Our environment is shaped not by human need but by business enterprise. Take the profit and hang the people. In the race for money, some men may come first, but Man comes last. Deserts are creeping up, and soil erosion is progressing by leaps and bounds. For profit forests are tumbled and fertilizers crumbled into our soil, depriving it of life and moisture, the essential ingredients for fertile land. Living more and more by the priorities of possessions, positions, and purse, we in this world have ceased to look beyond them.

Advertisers, whether of soda pop or streptomycin or LSD, know a lot of basic things about people, and they deliberately try to create a certain image in order to sell their products. How many of you have fallen for the tobacco habit which makes the smoker of a certain brand of cigarettes appear mature? Forget what Hugh Downs said about selling and education. He may really believe that "the promotion of good products is a form of education and a form that serves truth in the same way as promotion of an ethical ideal", but the majority of advertisers don't.

For years now advertisers have been conditioning us not only to buy certain things, but to live and think and aspire in certain ways. They realize the powers they have, but do you? The power I mean is the power to affect, deeply and lastingly, the nature, attitudes, and aspirations of millions of people.

On the business level these ways have been largely good. On the human and spiritual or moral level, I am not at all sure they are. I am now, of course, referring to a misleading and deceptive view of life and people that could, in the long run, be detrimental to mankind as a whole. Hence, the concern of Natural Hygiene and this book is to teach you to think out things for yourselves and lead the way by example rather than precept. For it is not enough to show people how to live better; there is a mandate for any group with powers of communication to show people how to be better. The two are not incompatible, but they can be divorced, and they are being divorced by the foolish images of how mankind lives that we see day in and day out on the T.V. screen or on the pages of the glossy magazines.

We would doubt whether there has been any time when a society was provided with fewer charts to the regions of behaviour, judgement, and choice than now, especially in the field of health, disease, and well being of man.

Nobody dares give you—our young ones—a compass because compasses, we are informed, are obsolete. True worth is where anyone wants to go; truth, in fact, is where you find it—a private enterprise.

So here we are, in a technological age, confronted with all sorts of things in all spheres of life, with no way to measure them except in terms of success and popularity, and even these are often inflated far beyond reality by press or clique support.

What we have arrived at is a kind of anarchy. Continuity, the solace of man, has been deliberately fractured, as windows are smashed by the attention-getters and the seekers—infantile and primitive—of instant gratification (instant art, instant sex, instant health, instant fame—it doesn't matter what you want as long as you get it now). How to dismiss these for what they are, still recognize the long-distance runners, the torch bearers, the real inheritors and innovators? Where is the dowser, divining the true creative springs of health and happiness? For sorely we need one: guide, compass, chart, call it what you will, to make at least a little sense out of what is close to chaos. Without it true civilization is merely a word and not a condition. Natural Hygiene and all that it stands for is one sort of a compass.

As to how you can make a clear pattern out of so many intangibles, including that greatest one—the very private I—it is fairly obvious.

The more you read and see and hear, the more equipped you will be to practice the art of association which is the basis of all understanding and judgment. The more you live and the more you look, the more aware you become of a consistent pattern underlying everything. Such a vein of consistency you will find in Natural Hygiene if you will only explore it with an open, unconditioned mind. You will soon then find out how much drug taking is fashion, how much is merely reflection.

We are frozen in this massive resistance to change, a resistance to any ideas which might, ironically, give our system the flexibility it needs to survive in a world of change. Are you, the young, going to perpetuate this doctrine of atrophy? Must you do the same thing for the sake of conformity, to follow the crowd, to be in with the group? Or are you, for the sake of your own future and your own country and for your children-to-come, going to ask some questions and demand some straightforward answers?

Much is required of those who answer them: reason, courage, and scrupulous honesty, but more than anything else, an open mind and an open heart. The generous can make trouble by giving away what they should sell. Natural Hygiene, by giving you your freedom instead of selling it to you, is freeing you from the shackles of that phrase: "One man's mediocrity is another man's good business".

Well may you ask: "How can we alter the state of things so that the undercurrent, 'Is it good?' becomes more powerful than the superfluous overflow, 'How much will it bring?' "

On you, the young generation, rests the task of protecting the inner sanctuary of conscience and creation from the intruders who come between the search and the truth.

Brave individuals are needed amongst you to tell your colleagues what is being done to them without their knowledge: the exploitation of eager interest and groping for truth by the muck-publishing merchants, the destruction of our natural environment and honest wholesome food by the chemical polluters, the exploitation of our fears and illness by drug marketers and would-be healers and sellers of "therapeutic modalities".

There are, however, still some individuals with integrity around. Your task is to draw the attention of your fellow beings to them—to those publishers of books and papers and magazines who put truth above expedience and the reader's needs ahead of the seller's market. You can start this by telling them about this book, about "Dr. Shelton's Hygienic Review", and the British publication, "The Hygienist".

It is such work and such people who must be supported if any balance is to be restored between the temporal and the spiritual, between commerce and communion, between guts of goodness and gold; and you must keep shouting for a higher standard of thinking, together with a better standard of living.

You youngsters, full of guts, gold, and gonads, will you buy this one from us? Help yourself and your friends to solve this awful problem. Make them aware that there is another way to be turned on and without drugs. Reorientate yourself to a constructive way of life.

As to those of us who are not in our teens and twenties, do we understand or try to understand the meaning of "turning on" and the revolution of the young? What is the significance of the expression "turned on"? It is ordinarily used by people for those who are under the influence either of drugs or of "pop" groups. We must understand it in a wider sense—to denote any process which people utilize to seek a more meaningful existence, whether by exploring hidden layers of the personality or enjoying new kinds of sensations ordinarily kept from them by habit or convention. Both habit and convention have played a tremendous part in stulitfying the spirit of "joie de vivre", health, and well-being in our young.

But the question remains: Why? Is the present vogue for "turning on", with its implications that there is something fundamentally wrong—"turned off" in fact—about our day-to-day living, simply a passing craze? Or does it reflect something of deeper significance—the beginnings of a revolution against a society which has shown itself unable to provide us with emotional, let alone spiritual, fulfilment?

To answer it honestly, we must take a peek at the history of turning on, as it has emerged from the work of the anthropologists. In its simplest and commonest form, it is a self-preservatory device evolved to protect the health of the human species.

In the days of old at the beginning of the emergence of men as homo sapiens, instinct performed this task, as it still does for animals in their wild state. They know, for example, what to eat, and what to avoid eating; they are rarely poisoned except, directly or indirectly, by man. They even instinctively preserve balance in what they eat—for example, fresh green pasture at one time and hay and corn at other times. Domesticated animals are less well protected by instinct; but research has shown that sheep are still capable of realizing which pasture contains all the requisite trace elements to keep them healthy, and of disregarding alternatives that to the human eye look more lush.

Man, however, as his conscious mind developed, began to lose these instincts—or, rather, the channel through which they had exercised their authority ceased to be available to him. Instinct had worked in animals by messages passed direct, as it were, to the muscular system. Instinct and action were synonymous. But with the attainment of reasoning, however, man gradually shed this type of control or suppressed it.

But the snag arose, when awareness took charge, cutting the old communications between instinct and the muscular system. There was no adequate provision made for an alternative telegraphic system to relay instinct's signals. They were passed to the unconscious mind, but it had no reliable way to make the conscious mind aware of their presence, let alone of their importance. It was to resolve this difficulty that turning on was first employed. There were always some individuals whose unconscious minds remained in charge (because they lived close to nature and in tune with nature), allowing the promptings of instinct to come through. The rest of the tribe began to be dependent on them for information which their own lost instinct could have given them, and the beginning of a cult was born.

In olden days music and dancing were greatly relied on to bring man close to nature and his own lost instincts. There was some sort of rapport between this feeling of "joie de vivre" that man experienced and the activity of singing and dancing. In this natural activity man forgot himself, lost his newly acquired inhibitions, and experienced, even if temporarily, that joy in sheer living.

The further he drew away from nature, the further he drew away from that very buoyancy of life which was the essence of his existence.

What we think of as the personality is often no more than society's imprint; underneath there is another one, dissatisfied with the world, waiting and wanting an opportunity to smash its way out.

Man wanted to recapture what he had lost. Since he could not define this "akin to nature" feeling, this buoyancy of well being and perpetual health and wholesomeness, he groped for it through devious ways.

Turning on, in fact, was, and remains, the standard device of primitive man to find himself and his well being. It is based on the fact that we are naturally healthy and would remain so if instinct was allowed to guide us; but because we have cut ourselves off from instinct's control, we need occasionally to be thrown back to it, as it were, for a quick overhaul. Just as singing and dancing shook up the mind and body before leaving both in a state of healing relaxation, so some such method of shocking ourselves back to nature was the beginning of an attempt to be turned on.

The great majority of people who present themselves for turning on do so out of a feeling that their old way of life is unsatisfactory, and a hope that they will feel their way to a new one.

For them drugs or any other orthodox "therapeutics", so-called, are not so much wrong as utterly irrelevant. As we have written in previous pages, the trouble is that society obviously needs this particular revolution—the breaking out by the young from a way of life that is failing them—and, for that matter, failing their elders.

It is not going to be easy, or safe—a revolution of this kind never is; but it is going to happen—or if it doesn't, there may be something much more destructive awaiting our society. The young person feels isolated because he no longer senses that he is part of the whole flow of life. A sense of wholeness, which healthy men and healthy societies have, is missing in the urban culture of America, Britain, and most other developing countries. Everything—man and his world—is fractured, compartmentalized, and contradictory. Countries like America, Britain, France, and Japan have never been so rich, yet poverty is an ever more stubborn and divisive condition.

Never has so much material comfort been available to so many, yet millions find life too hard to bear without daily tranquillizers or stimulants. "Civil liberties", so called, are expanding, yet imaginative and intelligent people are complaining that their chance to contribute to society creatively is shrinking. The more life is compartmentalized, the more do people write, talk, and study the subject of creativity. And the more the preoccupation with creativity grows, the less do many people feel it as part of the daily flow of their lives.

This hunger for being whole, holy, and healthy is aggravated by a growing awareness by young and old alike that the entire social and political structure is somehow out of control.

This hunger needs to be assuaged, and drugs won't do it. Natural Hygiene, if given a chance, can bring it about.

CHAPTER III

The Lesson of Thalidomide

"Will the next eighty years continue the downward plunge towards disaster, which has characterized the latter half of my life, or will mankind see the abyss ahead and turn back into a happier landscape? . . . man has survived hitherto because his ignorance and incompetence have made his folly ineffective. Now that science has shown us how to make folly effective, we must abandon folly or perish". (Bertrand Russell, on his 80th birthday).

The Thalidomide children will always be handicapped, though intensive efforts are now being made to help them lead as normal lives as possible. But the question remains— Are human guinea pigs justified as a means of sacrifice to maintain and regain health?

We feel that enough sacrifice has already been made by both animals and humans at the altar of so-called "medical science".

The responsibility of a doctor is primarily to teach his patients the means of maintaining and regaining their health. The word Doctor means a teacher—but we find no such teachings in the orthodox conception of health, disease, and healing.

The possibility that, in the future, outrageous conduct by perverted powers and acquiescent doctors may occur cannot, alas, be discounted; and the recent advances in pharmacology—the development of mind drugs in particular—as well as future discoveries that are bound to take place, allow us to envisage the existence of a situation whose nightmare aspects could make even the Thalidomide tragedy pale into insignificance.

That experimenting with new and various forms of drugs goes on ceaselessly and that human guinea pigs are involved, is not realized by the lay public. But in 1965, five years after the Thaliodomide disaster, human guinea

37

pig experiments were performed in Brooklyn, New York. Highly qualified medical specialists had injected liver cancer cells into debilitated patients without their consent or knowledge. One of these specialists was an expert on cancer and virology and a consultant to the United States Public Health Service. The research doctors were found guilty of unethical conduct, and the investigatory committee recommended that their medical licenses be suspended.

Dr. Henry Beecher of Harvard, writing in the New England Journal of Medicine (June 16, 1966), revealed further abuses of clinical medical experimentation. He told of 11 children who had their thymus glands removed while undergoing surgery for congenital heart disease. The thymectomies were proposed as part of a long-range study of "the growth and development of these children over the years". Dr. Beecher also gave many other documented examples of dubious experimental procedures.

Not all such "pure" experiments come to the knowledge of the public. In the great teaching hospitals some avantgarde doctors allow their scientific enthusiasm to outrun ethical considerations.

Sir Henry Ogilvie, consultant to Guy's London teaching hospital, writes: "What is new in medicine is research by fraud. The performance on patients (who have come to us in good faith for the cure of their ailments) of any number of tests and investigations, many of them unpleasant, some of them dangerous, all of them unnecessary for the diagnosis or treatment of their ailments . . ."

A Harley Street doctor, Mr. H. Pappworth, has made a point of airing publicly human guinea pig experiments in London teaching hospitals. In the British periodical "The Twentieth Century" he pointed out various experiments, notably one of large doses of ammonium chloride given to patients with liver diseases, producing profound neurological and psychological disturbances, varying from mild delirium to acute mania with frightening hallucinations.

Many readers will be appalled by the clinical experiments related above. Yet some of them may already have taken part unwittingly in a drug experiment. Many adults, at one time or another, have been prescribed a new drug. They have assumed it to be safe—their doctors know no better. They know it has first been tried out on laboratory animals, and that no untoward effects have been reported following the usual clinical trials. Although exhaustive short-time research is done, confidence cannot always be justified, however; from time to time national catastrophies occur, involving the health and life of the public. The Salk Polio Vaccine, when first introduced into the U.S.A., was a case in point. The Thalidomide disaster was another.

By 1960 Thalidomide, under the trade name of Couter-gan, had become the favourite sleeping tablet of West Germany. It could even be bought over the counter without a prescription. It has been combined with aspirin and other well-known drugs so that it could be taken for symptoms of nervousness, headaches, coughs, and colds. It was given by doctors to many patients, including pregnant women who were not sleeping well. Why not? The medical profession had always believed that health could be got out of a bottle, and that giving of drugs was like providing one of the amenities of life. They, of course, are under the same self-delusion that drugs "cure", like the rest of their patients.

The animal tests had been performed on mice, rats, guinea pigs, rabbits, etc., and the clinical trials had been most reassuring. The experimental stage of Thalidomide was then for practical purposes, over, since the pharmaceutical company responsible for manufacturing the sedative was sure of its safety.

For four years the company marketed Thalidomide in West Germany, and the results confirmed their confidence in the drug. They were successful in masking the symptoms. Indeed, a number of adults and children, either purposely or inadvertently, had taken overdoses of the drug, sometimes large overdoses. The suicide attempts were unsuccessful; the accidental overdoses led to some children sleeping for 16 hours, but they eventually recovered from their stupor. Thalidomide appeared to have a very low toxicity.

Then in 1960 a new clinical syndrome appeared, the outstanding feature of which was phocomelia (seal extremities). In other words, newborn children exhibited arms so short that their hands began almost directly from their shoulders. To a lesser degree, their legs showed defects of growth. There were also other congenital malformations. Phocomelia is rare, so rare that the majority of doctors never see a case during a lifetime of practice; but by the end of 1961 an epidemic of phocomelia had occurred in West Germany. Soon they tumbled on to the fact that phocomelia occurred in children born to mothers who had taken Thalidomide (made under the trade name of Contergan) in the early part of their pregnancy. In West Germany alone, 5900 Thalidomide babies were born. In Japan some 700 cases were reported by May, 1962; in Britain 430. Throughout the world, in fact, wherever Thalidomide was marketed under different trade names by different pharmaceutical companies, limbless and deformed children were born.

As we have seen in previous chapters, the Pill and the drug LSD are both suspects for causing almost the same kind of trouble in newborn babies. Yet trials go on, and the physician, ever believing in the miracle of drugs, goes boldly on.

The public may well ask whether tests on drugs by the pharmaceutical companies extend over a long enough period to establish the range of their so-called usefulness and their toxicity. If the answer is in the negative, then all those who take drugs are inadvertently participating in a human guinea pig experiment.

Dr. William Bean of the Iowa State University has said, in relation to the marketing of drugs: "The richest earnings occur when a new variety or variation of a drug is marketed before competing drugs can be discovered, improvised, named, and released. This bonanza time may last only a few months. Unless there are large earnings—the quick kill with the quick pill—the investment does not pay off. Commercial secrets must be kept dark, lest a competitor gets the jump. Under this system, it is impractical to do tests extending over a long period of months or years to establish the range of usefulness and potential dangers from toxicity. Such tests usually have to be done in hospitals and often in medical schools, where secrecy in science cannot be tolerated. Thus, after extensive laboratory tests on toxicity and pharmaceutical properties, but sometimes with a minimum of clinical trials, a drug may be marketed".

Thus the ethical position of the pharmaceutical companies, as well as the doctor, needs redefining. It is time the public was aware of the relationship between the profit motive of such firms and the dispensation of drugs to all and sundry, for this state of affairs needs a closer look.

The excuse by the medical profession that, how were they to know whether a drug given at the time of pregnancy can affect a foetus, is a lamentable excuse, as we shall show.

The protection of an unborn child by nature is a complicated effort. The child is enveloped in a heavy layer of membrane that does the job of filtering out any harmful substances present in the maternal blood and preventing it, as far as possible, from reaching the unborn child. However, there are many drugs (a fact well known to physicians) that do manage to evade this barrier and get through to the foetus.

How many miscarriages, abortions, and stillbirths are due to such drug poisoning? It is not just a matter of doubt that many babies are affected by drugs taken by the mothers before birth. For example, quinine taken by the mother is known to cause deafness and blindness in babies.

Babies are also poisoned after their birth when mothers continue to take the drug and suckle their child. The same applies to drugs in the milk of goats, cows, or other animals on whose milk the child is fed. Nicotine is found in the milk of mothers who indulge in smoking. DDT and penicillin are now found in the milk of goats and cows. Similarly, we can suspect that many other drugs find their way into the milk and eventually, to the child. It has long been suspected that alcohol imbibing in the mother gives the child a kind of stupor (drunkenness) and a tendency towards alcohol addiction. The same applies to young nicotine addicts via the smoke-laden atmosphere in a house, with a young baby inhaling such putrid air all the time. In many homes this is a number one air pollution going on.

It is now a well-established fact that narcotic substances do get through the natural filter (placenta) to the foetus. Nicotine and alcohol are both narcotics, and we must ask the question: How much of these two poisons affect the unborn babe?

As long ago as January 1956, the issue of the American Journal of Obstetrics and Gynaecology of that month carried an article by Drs. M. J. Goodfriend, M.D., I. A. Shey, M.D., and M. D. Klien, M.D., describing their observations of the effects of maternal narcotic addiction on the newborn, in which they show that narcotic addiction in the baby is a definite "clinical entity". They also show that the "abstinence symptoms" which occur in adult addicts, when they are denied their usual narcotics, also appear in the baby, when it is severed from the maternal supply. They tell us that the "neonatal abstinence syndrome" (complex of abstinence symptoms in the newborn) is uncommon, although they think that it is more common than the number of reported cases indicates.

If this is not an admission that the medical profession knew more than four years ago before the Thalidomide disaster that cases of narcotic addiction in the newborn of mothers who have been addicts do occur, what is?

In their studies they exchanged notes with other obstetricians and pediatricians, and were able to uncover ten cases of pregnancy "complicated" by drug addiction, while a search through medical literature yielded reports of 216 infants born to mothers who were drug addicts, during the period from 1892 to 1950. Of course, 190 babies showed symptoms of addiction, and 26 showed no symptoms as such. They state that the babies who developed post-natal symptoms showed a characteristic "abstinence syndrome". They point out that most of the physicians reporting such cases tell of the normal appearance of infants at birth, but within twenty-four to seventy-two hours there appears a progressive restlessness and irritability, accompanied by shrill crying, which may continue for hours and gives the impression that the infant is in pain.

Can anyone now doubt that the medical profession was not innocent about the Thalidomide disaster? Did they not have evidence here that poisons, narcotics, drugs, call them what you will, can get through to the foetus and affect its behaviour and possibly therefore, its structure? What more evidence was needed than that the babies feed poorly and commonly vomit the little food that is taken by mouth? Such other symptoms as yawning, intermittent cyanosis (blueness of lips and skin from lack of oxygen), diarrhoea, lacrimation (tearing), diaphoresis (sweating), and salivation (excessive flow of saliva), severe dystrophy (faulty nourishment), occur, with the infant sometimes dying in convulsions, are enough evidence for anyone sane enough to sit up and take notice, of the harmfulness of such poisoning. These authors say that as a general rule the symptoms of narcotic addiction in the newborn resemble the "Abstinence Syndrome" seen in adults. Such a syndrome is a state of partial collapse following the withdrawal of alcohol, opiates, or stimulants.

We ask, why did they not tell the public of their findings? Why did they not warn all mothers and mothers-to-be about the effects of taking poisons in their bodies? Some of their statements concerning the addiction of mothers indicate that these mothers had been made into drug addicts by their very physicians who administered narcotics to relieve pain, an ancient procedure that is resorted to by those practitioners who refuse to give any consideration to cause. Suppressing pain, no matter how, leads to more pain and more "need" for suppression.

Casting out the Devil with Beelzebub is a practice that is old and honoured among the medical fraternity. The Thalidomide disaster is the price that was paid—not by them—but by innocent children and gullible people who trusted that "experts" know best.

It is the practice of the medical profession to blame congenital deformities and weakness on heredity. This inheritance factor is tremendously overplayed in importance and incorrectly blamed for the tragedies encountered in births and infant life.

Thalidomide, under the trade name of Distaval, was marketed in Britain in 1959/1960 and very soon afterwards, reports appeared which seemed to indicate its use with the causation of peripheral neuritis. Patients using it as a sleep inducer found that the tips of their fingers or their toes felt numb; or they complained of pins and needles, or of pain or weakness in their limbs.

This side effect of Distaval was a topic discussed fully in an article by Drs. Pamela Fullerton and Michael Kramer of Middlesex Hospital in the British Medical Journal of September 30, 1961.

Then again in the issue of October 21, 1961, the same British Medical Journal published a letter with some case histories from Whipps Cross Hospital, the writer going so far as to suggest that Thalidomide appeared to be "fast becoming one of the commonest causes of neuropathy in neurological clinics". At the same time the British Medical Journal allowed advertisement for Distaval to appear in its pages, making no mention of side-effects, but on the other

hand, allowing the advertisement to be concluded in a misleading manner thus—"There is no case on record in which
even gross overdosage with Distaval has had harmful results. Put your mind at rest. Depend on the safety of
Distaval".

Thus, in spite of the warming by Fullerton and Kramer
that "some evidence that abnormalities are not confined to
the peripheral nervous system" and that several observers
suggested, when seeing some of those patients before
Thalidomide toxicity was suspected, that the clinical features of these cases resembled those of neuropathy associated with malignant disease, the drug was not taken off
the market.

The tragedy of Thalidomide was thus due to the blind
obstinacy of those who weighed their pecuniary gain
against the welfare of the patients. This was proved when
Dr. Frances Kelsey of the U.S. Food and Drug Administration persuaded the F.D.A. to delay the introduction of
Thalidomide in the U.S.A., much to the irritation of the
manufacturers, Merrell, who had acquired the rights to it.
As a result, Dr. Kelsey came in for some abuse, even in
Britain. However, she was right in her surmise that the
symptoms of peripheral neuritis, though trivial in themselves, are often a reflection of more serious disorder.

The pretext and excuses that the medical profession was
not aware of any harm from Thalidomide and hence, was
freely given, does not hold water and is not valid under the
circumstances. Clearly, the medical profession has fallen
into the trap that lies in wait for all guilds: it has grown
self-indulgent, losing the capacity for self-criticism.

Natural Hygiene has always—and within the past few
years the epidemiologists of the medical profession have
also—realized that most congenital (resulting from one's
heredity) deformities are not foreordained by heredity, but
are preventable accidents of development in the womb.
It is very possible to circumvent most congenital deformities by improving the preparation for pregnancy and by
careful attention to stresses and to Natural Hygiene habits
during this period.

Many do not realize that both the embryo (the develop-
mental stage until three months) and foetus (the develop-
mental stage from three months to birth) are subject to the

action of the elements and malice of the mother's non-hygienic living habits.

These symptoms go unnoticed at the time; they may be signalled only by a rash, occasional headaches, vomiting, bad temper, or nervousness. For often there is no sign of the tragedy until the baby is born with a single eye (cyclopia) or a dwarfed body, a cleft palate, unhearing ears, unseeing eyes, a blighted mind, cataracts, monstrosities, heart disease, or with heart and organs being left outside the chest cavity, or in failure of one or both legs or arms to develop, or in erythroblastosis fetalis.

Experiments on animals, and Hygienists disdain this practice, have demonstrated conclusively that crippling deformities arise from injuries and irritations to the embryo at certain stages of its development. An embryo that began its life with perfectly normal "genes" may, by the time it is born, have only one eye, or two heads, or three legs. External stresses applied to these animals included feeding deficient diets, subjection to extremes of temperature, putting them through mazes and tunnels to unnerve and perplex them, diminution of oxygen, reduction of sufficient sleep and rest, and other things to produce enervation. Effects of like disturbances and adverse influences on human beings (pregnant women) have been proved beyond doubt.

The results that ensue from the foregoing insults to the unborn baby depend on the time they occur or the time that their cumulative poisonous effect has reached beyond the danger point of toleration. It is possible to draft a time table or calendar which relates deformities to the age of the embryo at the time of injury or passing the vital toleration point of accumulated toxic materials. The latter are caused by the incorrect mode of living and consumption of drugs.

For example, stresses producing a one-eyed baby generally may come during the first week or two after fertilisation of the egg for at this time the cellular parts from which the two eyes will develop are so close together as to be virtually single.

Next in order comes the stage at which conjoined (Siamese) twins may originate from an injury which prevents separation of the two individuals. In about the third week critical injury or "toleration toxins" may result in the heart or other organs being left outside the body cavity, or maldevelopment of legs or arms may occur because this is the time when the heart and viscera are still outside the body cavity and the limbs are formed and starting to grow. Injury in the fourth week, when the windpipe is developing from the gullet, may produce the well-known defect which leaves an opening between the windpipe and gullet—tracheo-oesophageal fistula.

In the fifth week, when the lenses of the eye are forming, the embryo is vulnerable to congenital cataract. During the seventh week it may be doomed to a cleft palate for the separated two halves of the palate normally start to close at this period. Injury or toxic accumulation in the eighth week may produce mongolism. It is at this point that the embryo begins to develop the base of the brain and skull, the wall of the heart, the nasal bones, and the fingers—all structures that are blighted in mongolism.

The inner ear undergoes rapid differentiation during the ninth week, and a mishap at this stage may result in a deaf baby. This is only part of the list of defects that can be created at the respective ages of the embryo, and the whole matter rsets on quite a more or less orderly, scientific basis.

All this the pushers of drugs knew. They were well aware of the consequences that could occur. The question arises whether the Thalidomide disaster would have been averted if the drug had first been tested on pregnant laboratory animals. Various scientists have made post hoc tests on Thalidimide in this way. *Investigations on such animals as mice and hamsters did not yield convincing results.* With other species though—the New Zealand white rabbit, for example—specific doses of Thalidomide, administered during a definite period in pregnancy, led to limb deformities in the newborn of offspring, similar to those seen in human babies. Clearly then, drug testing in animals is not only unnecessary but ineffective. The fact remains that, despite animal tests and human clinical trials, no drug is absolutely safe.

Most of these deformities can be prevented, and congenital abnormalities that have appalled and frightened mankind since antiquity should become avoidable if humans would only realize that the health and development of the evolving foetus are based on every and any factor of life that affects the health and well being of the mother, either positively or negatively.

Thalidomide is, however, not the only drug that is now worrying the medical profession. One of the latest drugs to come under suspicion of having a teratogenic effect is one sold in England under the name Marzine. In use for more than a decade, it is prescribed for "motion sickness". The British manufacturers of the drug have issued a warning statement about the drug, in which they say: "Since the possibility tthat there may be some risk, however slight, cannot be entirely discounted, this statement is made at the earliest opportunity to advise against the use of this drug in early pregnancy".

Naturally after such a disaster, there is a growing distrust even among the medical profession of all drugs in early pregnancy, as will be apparent from the following warning issued by the medical journal The Lancet for March 23, 1963: "At present the use of any drug in pregnancy is rightly looked upon with uneasiness, and in view of the recent maternal death in which the prolonged use of predinsolone may have been a factor, I should like to question whether the giving or continuing of steroids in pregnancy is justifiable, except of course, in emergency . . . Of course, this policy, if strictly carried out, would mean that no patient of the childbearing age should ever be given steroids, but would this really be a serious loss to therapeutics"?

Hygienists would answer the last question with an unequivocal "No". You can see how the mind of a physician is always oriented towards drugs. The very word Physician means one learned in the art of drugging. Deprive the physician of his drugs and he flounders—because he has no conception of what health is and how to go about achieving it.

Teratogenesis is the development of a deformed foetus. A drug that tends to occasion fatal deformation is known to be teratogenic. As we have said before, there was considerable evidence that there were drugs that deformed the unborn, but the tendency was to ignore the fact and even to hide it. It was the Thalidomide disaster that brought the matter out into the open and compelled attention to that matter.

The medical profession had always insisted that few

teratogenic drugs result in serious side-effects in the mother.
This was not true of Thalidomide and is probably not true
of other drugs. We cannot expect that a drug that can de-
form an unborn baby would be harmless to the mother.

Before even the Thalidomide disaster, it was an established fact that both insulin and thyroid extract are
teratogenic. A great deal of work had gone in to show that
when mothers take these drugs during pregnancy, as many
as 70 percent of them experienced miscarriages or gave
birth to premature, malformed, or dead babies.

An unnamed British physician has been quoted as saying
that although "until recently the subject has been somewhat
neglected in clinical medicine, much work has been done in
experimental animals on the effects to the foetus of various
drugs given during pregnancy . . ." Can we not then ask
why it should take a major worldwide disaster before
physicians give heed to the knowledge already available?
Has science become such a God that the welfare of human
beings does not matter?

The same physician pointed out that certain drugs should
be avoided during the early stages of pregnancy and others
in the late stages, saying "It is particularly important to
avoid treatments during the first three months with any
hormone preparations which have (sex) effects, however
slight". The consequences of not heeding this warning may,
according to him, result in malformations of a masculine
character in female infants. What happens to male infants
he does not say.

Among the drugs to be avoided in the final stages of
pregnancy, he lists the sulfa drugs, barbiturates, and the
anti-coagulants. Thus the very drugs prescribed by the
physician to pregnant mothers (the barbiturates to enable
them to "sleep", and the anti-coagulants to prevent bleeding
at birth) are among the drugs that are likely to harm the
infant.

It is like closing the door after the horse has bolted when
we hear such statements like the following by eminent
physicians. J.D. Ebert, M.D., director of the Department
of Embryology of the Carnegie Institute, issued such a
warning saying: "Many of the staggering number of children now born each year with congenital defects—conservatively estimated at five percent—might be spared
lifelong misery and their parents spared endless distress if

the unborn were protceted against some of the new wonder drugs taken by their mothers during pregnancy . . . We must recognize that the chemistry and the physiology of the embryo are unique and that the current practice of testing new drugs only on adult animals offers no assurance that they are safe for administration during pregnancy".

Another question we could ask: How much of the mental retardation and minor congenital defects of children are due to drug-taking by mothers? Also: What effect does the giving of drugs to infants and young children have on their growth and development? It is well known that tobacco stunts both physical and mental development. How many other drugs do the same? When the babies in the Binghamton, N.Y. hospital received salt in their formulas and some of them were killed, it was asserted that it would be necessary to wait several years to determine how much mental damage the salt may have produced. It seems to be understood that salt can retard brain development.

The F.D.A. experimenters have admitted that: "It has been shown in the case of some antibiotics, hormones, and chemotherapeutics that there is a transmission of these compounds by the human placenta, and this raises the question of possible resultant toxic effects on the foetus".

They also admit that there is rapid transmission of some drugs and that the concentration of the drug in the foetal circulation may be high. For example, they admit that with tetracline the level of this drug in the foetal circulation has been shown to be as high as 75 percent of that in the mother's blood.

Once again we repeat—the solution to such problems can never be met by legislation or any kind of testing. There can be no safety ever. As an article in Topic (London) of December 1, 1962 said: "Every drug, if it is to be effective, is potentially dangerous". An English physician and surgeon, Harry Lillie, M.D., says: "Modern-day drugs are completely useless and even dangerous". We agree with him and say that all drugs, modern and old ones, are useless and damaging. The only safe, sane, and sensible solution to prevent another Thalidomide tragedy is to abolish all drugs, for so-called "curative" purposes.

The latest report to come out in the press is against our old friend Aspirin—Aspirin has been regarded all these years as one of the safest drugs. Now we read in the San

Antonio Star (an American newspaper) of October 26, 1975 the following headlines: "Aspirin Danger to Expectant Mothers". In this report they say that taking of aspirin during pregnancy can cause delivery problems, haemorrhaging and anaemia. These studies were carried out in Australia by two of the most respected doctors in that country. The two doctors, Edith Collins anl Gillian Turner, based their report on intensive studies of 144 women.

They reported: The regular consumption of aspirin was detrimental to the health of these patients during pregnancy and to the welfare of their babies."

The women under study were divided into two groups: the first group, rated as "constant takers" of aspirin were allowed to remain on a daily diet of aspirins; the second group were only allowed to consume one aspirin a week. The results were dramatic:

1) Women in the first group, the regular users, showed they were twice as likely to develop anaemia as the second group.

2) They exhibited a haemorrhage rate four times higher than the second group.

3) They had four times higher incidence of late delivery. Both doctors admitted that chronic aspirin users run a greater risk of losing their child than non-users. They also came to the conclusion that aspirin addicts run a greater risk of having a smaller child.

And yet the medical profession doled out billions of tons of Aspirin to the world at large as if they were "goodies" and could do no harm. This has been going on for nearly 150 years.

Dr. Reba M. Hill, Associate Professor of Pediatrics at Baylor College of Medicine in Houston, Texas, U.S.A., admitted that 60 percent of pregnant women took aspirin during pregnancy; also that there were traces of aspirin levels that could be identified in 40-50 percent of newborn infants.

As long as the art of drugging is practised, another disaster like Thalidomide is bound to take place sooner or later. The only way to avoid it is to teach healthful living habits and an abhorrence of all drugs to our children and grandchildren.

· CHAPTER IV

Drugs Cannot Heal You

"I declare, as my conscientious conviction, founded on long experience, and reflection, that if there was not a single physician, surgeon, man-midwife, chemist, apothecary, druggist, nor drug, on the face of the earth, there would be less sickness and less mortality than now prevail."

Jas. Johnson, M.D., F.R.S.
Editor of The Medico-Surgical Review

For hundreds of years, drugs of all kinds have been used as "curative" agents in the treatment of disease. Millions of pounds and dollars are spent yearly in their production. Wonderfully equipped laboratores are established all over the world for experimental purposes in connection with the use of drugs, and a tremendous industry has grown up around their preparation and commercial exploitation. They have become almost an integral part of civilized life.

A drug may be defined as any substance, mineral, vegetable or animal, other than foodstuffs, that produces changes within the living structures and organs of the human system. In accepting this definition, we have to make an essential point quite clear: such changes as may be produced in the body are not the result of any active agency within the drug, but because of the vital response of the living tissues against the effect of the drug. If we keep this point in mind, it will help us to understand the valid objections which the Hygienist makes against their use.

The history of drugs, their discovery and use, would make a very long story. There is little doubt that the use of a great many of them originated as a result of a total misconception of the physiological disturbances which are at the back of every disease process. It is a well-established fact that, in the early history of mankind, all disorders of the body were regarded as dangerous to the life of the individual and largely the result of some evil influence. The taking of such substance brought about an immediate change in the symptoms of the disease process and it was naturally assumed that such a change was desirable. Thus, the search began for those agents which would bring relief from pain and change, or abate, the symptoms that accompanied physiological disturbances.

The time, thought, and labour that has been put into such a search has been prodigious. Every known substance has been experimented with in order to ascertain its so-called "curing properties" upon the human system in disease. With the quest for the substances that would "cure disease", it was natural that a great deal of superstitious belief would be associated. Every substance has been able to claim marvellous results at one time or another, and the folk lore of every people is full of stories relating to the cure of disease through various remedies and concoctions. As Draper says: "Mystical experimenters for centuries have ransacked all Nature, from the yellow flowers which are sacred to the sun, and gold, his emblem and representative on earth, down to the vilest excrements of the human body".

The sum total of the resultant knowledge from all these researchers represents pharmacology. The application of this knowledge represents, to a great extent, the present-day practice of medicine, and the whole scheme of producing and employing these agents in the treatment of disease is built upon no more secure foundation than the vaguest empiricism.

Dr. John Cowan, M.D., an enlightened medical doctor, admitted this when he wrote, "Drugs, no matter in what form, under what conditions, in what quantity, under what name, patented or otherwise, have been, are, and will continue to be, in proportion to their use, a great and positive curse to God's human family.

This great and almost universal delusion—namely, that by the taking of drugs or patent medicines a sick person can be restored to health, is shown in all its absurdity in the supposition that what will make a well person sick, will make a sick person well. This is a great fallacy, as is sadly shown by millions that have passed off from the earth's surface before half their days were spent. Since the creation of the world—or since the days of Hippocrates, if you will—drugs never have cured one single person having a disease of any nature. When it is asserted they have done so, it will be found on closer examination and argument that the person has recovered comparative health in spite of drugs and not through their influence."

Hygienists contend that healing is a biological process and not an art; that healing takes place because of the inherent instinct of the body to preserve itself in good health and efficiency. A Hygienist's approach to disease is the antithesis of the medical. We seek not to fool the patient by masking symptoms with drugs, but we give the patient all the normal requisites of life in accordance with his needs and capacities; we eliminate the cause of his troubles and, above all, he is accorded a physiological rest which have been wasted by enervating habits.

Drugs are not needed and are not used in a state of health. They have no normal or physiological relation to the body. If taken orally or intravenously in a state of health, they are eliminated as rapidly as the excretory organs can expel them. Neither are they needed in a state of disease and are also eliminated as rapidly as the sick organism can dispose of them. The relation of a poison to the body does not become changed or altered because the body is sick. A drug loses none of its toxicity because the body is sick. It actually prolongs the disease because the organism recognises the nature of the drug and immediately begins the process of eliminating the drug as fast as possible and, in doing this, the disease for which it was taken seems to get better because the symptoms are temporarily alleviated. The organism cannot do two things at once and do them equally well. An emergency has arisen, and it has to forget the lesser toxic state and deal with the drug, but after the drug has been excreted, the organism once again manifests the symptoms of disease for which the drug was taken. The drug itself had added to the toxic load, and often more and varied symptoms than the original are manifested so that the 'cure' becomes worse than the disease. This causes the disease process to be unnecessarily prolonged, and if the patient is very weak it may prevent him from ever recovering. The energy of the patient should be used in getting well and should not be wasted in fighting drugs, foreign agents, or other so-called treatments which only interfere with the effort of the body in setting itself right. That the body has the power for self-repair can be observed in the case of the healing of a wound. That "nature alone heals" is as true today as it was when living organisms came into being.

Even orthodox physicians are beginning to pay lip service to this well-established fact. The Washington Daily News (August 16, 1960) carried an item by John Troan under the heading, "Doctors called too fast with Pen and Needle", in which he quotes some revealing statements made by Joost Meerloo, M.D., psychiatrist of Colombia University, in an article in the journal The American Practitioner. Meerloo complains that physicians often reach too quickly for their pens or needles, meaning they are in too much of a hurry to write a prescription or to inject a drug. As this is not news to Hygienists, we naturally wonder why it has taken so long for him to make the discovery. He points out that "nature" takes care of a lot of ills, if given a chance—for every organism is equipped with "spontaneous regenerative forces". "Nature" here would appear to mean the organism's own restorative and self-healing capacity. He goes further, declaring that physicians "give themselves very little opportunity to observe and evaluate these spontaneous healing forces in the patient". He adds that, instead, physicians are over-anxious "to do something and to interfere with processes we know so little about". This is an indictment as bad as that given by Sir William Osler, "We put medicines of which we know little in bodies of which we know even less".

We Hygienists have always maintained that, if Natural Hygiene had to oppose drug therapy purely on its intrinsic value in recovery from disease, its task would be relatively easy, but there is another driving force behind the production of drug remedies which adds a further important dimension to the mater. A headline in The Medical News, January 26, 1968, "Drugs Give Top Profits" reminds us of this fact. The figures which are given come from the United States where, it seems, an investigation into drug prices is now going on. Dr. Miller cited a study of relative investment returns made in 1966 of a cross-section of American businesses: drugs and medicines led, giving a stockholder a return of 21.1 percent—more than investment in periodicals (20.1); radio and television equipment (19.8); motor vehicles (17.1); and computing machines (16.3). He was testifying before a Monopoly Subcommittee, as part of Senator Gaylord Nelson's investigations into drug pricing.

Not only do chemists sell drugs to physicians for daily use in the treatment of minor and serious diseases, but they are sold direct to the consumer for use at his own discretion. Of course, certain highly and immediately dangerous drugs are sold under close scrutiny, but the public can still get at them through prescriptions from physicians. The public still appears to be willing to be fooled by the promises of cures and their credulity is certainly not left unexploited.

But, while drugs have no power to cure ,they do possess the power to destroy. This is a point that so few know anything about. When people take cathartics and laxatives, they do not realize how much damage they do to the membranes of the bowel. They may be sugar or chocolate coated and deceive the palate, but their irritation will exact a toll later on. The constant irritation which they induce will often produce congestion, inflammation and, finally, morbid changes in the membranes. Then sufferers who are told that they have colitis, proctitis, appendicitis, haemorrhoids, or some other complaint, will never think that the so-called simple remedies are to blame. Another result of taking such things is that other organs like the kidneys and the liver may be directly affected. The irritating substances set up inflammatory processes there and in various other organs as well, and the first stage may be the onset of some serious and chronic disease.

Gallons of drugs are taken as tonics. In most cases mineral iron is used for this purpose. It is a well-known fact that it will destroy the teeth, but few realize that it continues this destructive effect throughout the system. The alimentary tract is affected by contracting the tissues and causing constipation; this drug (iron) irritates the bladder and will set up changes there that may lead to all kinds of after-effects. Quinine is another drug that many take at odd times, without realizing its potency and the harm it does. They may take it in the first stage of a feverish cold, unmindful of the fact that it will do much more damage than the actual cold. Text books tell us that its frequent use will lead to one or more of the following conditions: ringing in the ear, heaviness in the head, disturbances of vision, colour blindness, irritation of the kidneys and stomach, the passing of blood in the urine, neurasthenia, skin eruptions and debility.

One could go on citing drug after drug, but we hope to show such procedures used in simple and serious illnesses have ultimately a devastating effect upon the whole body.

If we object to this method of treating disease, what alternatives or substitutes have we to offer for recovery of health? If we understand the basic principles of Natural Hygiene, we know that abolition—not substitution—is required. We know that every living organsm is endowed by Nature with the inherent power to heal, repair, and recuperate. If we use our capacity to understand and leave Nature intelligently alone to do its job, instead of spending our time searching for new remedies and cures, the foundaton upon which drug experimentation is built would be quckly swept away. We should realise that most of the symptoms and bodily conditions for which drugs are ordinarily prescribed, are evidence of curative or self-cleansing efforts of the human system and that, if we administer drugs, we are actually laying the foundations of disease by checking or obstructing the regenerative forces of Nature.

Far from encouraging healing to take place, drugs are inherently inimical to the welfare of the body. A poison is a poison qualitatively and not quantitatively. Anything which cannot be classified as food and utilized by the living body for its welfare can be classed as a poison. Drugs cannot be utilized and incorporated into the living tissue as flesh and blood like an apple or nuts, hence can belong to no other classification but that of a poison.

It is an irony that perhaps the best commentary on drugs and orthodox medicine should come from an experienced medical practitioner, Dr. Ulric Williams, the original "Radio Doctor of New Zealand: "Medical 'Science' is not healing disease. Do we ever see cancer, tuberculosis, eczema, anaemia, paralysis, goitre, osteomyelitis, epilepsy, asthma, neurosis, insanity, or even the common cold healed by medical 'science'? We do not. Medical so-called 'science' is nothing but an arduous way of converting acute illnesses into chronic disease . . .

No-one has ever been cured of cancer by surgery and

nobody ever will; though victims climb over each other
for the privilege of being exterminated by what one hospital matron described as 'the senseless butchery that goes
on in our operating theatres . . .' Radium, X-Rays, drugs,
and surgery are nothing but clumsy, illogical, expensive,
and painful . . . techniques for shortening life and increasing misery."

Reality (16.5.47)

CHAPTER V

Drugs Are Poisons

"All our curative agents are poisons and, as a consequence, every dose diminishes the patient's vitality."

Prof. Alonso Clark, M.D.

That drugs are poisons and lethal according to their toxicity is a fact which even the medical profession cannot deny. Hygienists have always contended that there are no such things as safe drugs and that no amount of testing drugs on animals can make them safe for humans.

The validity of this is shown in the following quotation from Biochemistry by Kleener & Orkten (C.V. Mosby Co. St. Louis, U.S.A.) Page 888, 1966 edition: "Drugs tested on animals cannot be administered to the human being with absolute assurance of safety since detoxication routes may vary in different species (including the human being). Most detoxications occur in the liver."

The medical profession has often taken the credit (not rightly theirs) for the eradication of many so-called infectious diseases which were rampant once upon a time in Europe and America. In order to assure the "safety" of the population of the world, they have, from time to time, opened their Pandora's Box and urged us, the public, to be drugged, vaccinated, immunized, and injected by various poisons, promising us protection from germs, viruses, "infections", and such like in safety if not in comfort.

How safe are we? Has the so-called advance of medical science truly succeeded in stemming the tide? For this, one has only to look at the third report covering 1961-64, which the World Health Organization publishes every few years.

"As expected, it makes depressing reading. But this is not just because its cold figures represent such an appalling

58

sum of human misery. It also raises the spectre of an
endless, increasingly expensive and exhausting chase after
a dream figure called 'health', whom we shall never catch.
Above all, it hits hard at the euphoric faith that we have
only to develop the right miracle drug or vaccine and, with
a little effort, we can knock out infectious diseases for all
time". So says an article in the New Statesman, dated
May 27, 1966. The article then continues, "In fact, of
course, no infection is knocked out until the last molecule
of drug or vaccine that we shall ever need has strangled
the guts of the last germ in the last man in the last village.
This will always be totally impracticable, even in sophisticated societies (have you had all your polio jabs?) So
despite all the brave talk of 'total eradication'—a particular
failing of W.H.O.—one is back to control. There is no
real call for euphoria here either. One of the paradoxes of
the last 20 years has been that, with infection after infection
'conquered', the percentage of hospital beds occupied by
sufferers from infection is as high as it was 50 years ago.
The super-armoury of drugs, vaccines, and modern sanitation may diminish acute or semi-acute infections but it is
also uncovering a range of latent micro-organisms that can
now express themselves. Meanwhile the acute infections
are proving more difficult and costly to keep down.

Yaws is a nasty example. A few years ago the big
WHO/UNICEF campaign, which examined 150,000 people and injected 30,000 with a few pennyworths of long-
lasting penicillin, received worldwide publicity. It clearly
did an immense amount of immediate good, but now WHO
is expressing concern that Yaws seems to be reappearing
in 'treated' populations. Venereal disease, which the com-
placent might have thought had been controlled by penicillin in the 1950s, is now rampaging back to wartime
levels. Cholera has crashed back after its decline in the
1950s and, the report declares, is now 'an actual threat to
the health of the world'. El Tor cholera has appeared in
new areas and is spreading from its endemic area in the
Celebes Islands.

Smallpox, as we know in Britain, is very far from being
controlled. It also neatly illustrates the cost of control and
the self-deluding fantasy of eradication. This month the
19th World Health Assembly announced a 10-year programme to eradicate smallpox, to start next year. The

plan is to vaccinate the entire population (1,790,000) of the remaining endemic areas in Africa, S.E. Asia, and South America at a cost of $180,000. *There is every reason to believe, the WHO claim, that given nearly 100 percent coverage this programme "can rapidly 'eradicate' the disease".* (my italics) This optimism is based on the belief that there are no animal reservoirs or vectors for the disease—that it is transmitted only from human to human —and that permanent immunity in the great majority of the population should stop any spread. "Stop" in this context is a strong word. It gives the impression that once all those millions of needles have plunged in, we can relax. In fact, of course, the price of freedom is eternal and costly vigilance. In Europe and North America the price of "almost" complete freedom from smallpox is put at between $43 and $70 million a year.

Meanwhile an appalling list of diseases are being controlled only slowly, or hardly at all. Malaria is still the chief problem in many areas and, with increasing insecticide resistance and the vectors going into hiding in animal populations, it looks like a long—even an endless—battle. WHO claim that 444 million out of the 1,560,000 in malarious areas have been "liberated", while a further 723 million are covered by "eradication" programmes. In Africa, though, control has hardly begun; 'problems are great and the means are lacking'. Bilharziasis (snail fever) comes second as a cause of death and ill health. Control is proving difficult and disappointing, while 180 million to 200 million now have the disease. With trachoma, the greatest single cause of blindness, progress is more or less backwards. Ten years ago the number of victims was put at 400 million. Now, the Third Report indicates, more trachoma is being found in the increasing child population and groups not previously surveyed, while hopes for trachoma vaccines have not been realized. Sleeping sickness is also on the increase.

Meanwhile in the developed countries where infectious diseases have been "conquered", cardiovascular disease causes 40 percent of all deaths; accidents are now the leading killer of everyone under 35 in most countries; lung cancer is becoming a major hazard . . . The dream of Beveridge of "finding a health service which will diminish disease by prevention and cure", is still as far off as ever—as it will always be."

If it is on such weak foundations that the so-called science of medicine is offering us safety, is it not time to look somewhere else?

As recently as February 1, 1975 the medical journal The Lancet admitted that "McKeown et al. demonstrated that the decline in mortality in England and Wales, France, Hungary, Ireland and Sweden in the nineteenth century was almost entirely independent of direct medical intervention (and may even have occurred in spite of it) and was almost completely the result of better food and public health measures, such as the introduction of pure water supplies and the installation of adequate sewage systems. Razzell suggests that advances in personal hygiene were also probably very important".

One of the pioneers of Natural Hygiene, Dr. John Tilden, M.D. put forward a similar argument based on facts, way back in 1938 when he questioned the role of medicine in promoting the health and welfare of mankind.

A report in the London Times (June 24, 1975) commenting on an article on the subject of whooping cough and immunisation which appeared in the British Medical Journal, said: "Reductions in the numbers of babies vaccinated against whooping cough have had no effect on the number of cases of the disease notified. The total reported each week has declined steadily this year from a peak in the autumn of 1974, according to the Public Health Laboratory Service. In the past 10 years the level of the peak in each epidemic period has been getting lower; whereas 500 cases were reported in the peak weeks of 1974, the figure was about a thousand in 1970/1971."

The interesting thing about the various forms of immunisation is that, as history shows, the disease was already on the decline when immunisation was introduced. It has happened in the past with Diphtheria and Scarlet Fever and it is now happening with Whooping Cough.

A headline in Medical News (June 12, 1975) read: "Anti-Rheumatic drug deaths 'disquieting', proving once again the poisonous nature of these death-dealing chemicals introduced into the human body. The report went on to say:

"In a survey in which mortality rather than morbidity of drugs was studied, the number of deaths attributed to drug therapy is described by Dr. P.M. Brooks and his colleagues at the Centre for Rheumatic Diseases, Glasgow as "disquieting"."

How safe is safe, we ask, when the pharmacists and physicians themselves are not sure about the things they administer to their patients under the guise of "safe and sure treatment"?

This is what Dr. Cahal says in The Pharmaceutical Journal of March 27, 1966, "It must be clearly understood that no drug could ever be regarded as wholly safe for all patients. Anyone who expects to be able to take active drugs without any risks at all is expecting the impossible. The establishment of any controlling authority, whether it has legal powers or not, cannot make drugs 100 percent safe."

It seems that "safe" is a word that is loosely used by the drug industry when advertising their wares, when really they are well aware that they mean no such thing. The London Times of March 25, 1966, publishes a report on vaccination against measles and comes out with "there is little if any advantage in providing a child with a temporary protection against measles, only to allow him to develop it in later life when its effects tend to be much more serious than in childhood".

Dr. Alexis Carrel, generally accepted as a leading authority on modern medicine and a Nobel Prize Winner, has summed up our hygienic contentions for us in these words: "Medicine is far from having decreased human suffering as much as it endeavours to make us believe . . . the suppression of diphtheria, smallpox, typhoid fever, etc., are paid for by the long sufferings and the lingering deaths caused by chronic infections, and especially by cancer, diabetes, and heart disease". (Man The Unknown).

In another place he says, rather plaintively: "We should perhaps renounce this artificial form of health and exclusively pursue Natural Health".

If only people would try leaving their body intelligently alone and not suppress their symptoms with drugs, more than half the hospitals in the world would be emptied in no time at all.

A medical journal once remarked cynically that a new

drug should be used quickly before it has lost its effectiveness; with legislation on drugs, many old drugs have been declared obsolescent. As Dr. Shelton, the doyen of Natural Hygiene, has said many times, "the cures come and the cures go—but the curing goes on for ever".

As we have already said, drugs are derived from many sources, the inorganic world supplying us with alkalies, acids, metals, and other chemical compounds; and the organic world, through the vegetable kingdom, yields an enormous quantity of substances which are used in drugging practice. Many people, still deluded by sentimental folklore, imagine that vegetable drugs do not have the same potency as those derived from other sources; hence, the revival of "herbal remedies" and such like. However, some of the most virulent poisons are derived from the vegetable kingdom. The animal kingdom yields certain substances which are used as therapeutic agents, and these substances are being more extensively employed at the present time in what is known as "glandular" or hormone therapy".

Now, in order to understand the effects of drugs on the human system, we must know some physiology. The so-called 'physiological action" of drugs has no relationship to the normal physiology of a living body. All such effects belong to the realm of pathology.

When a certain substance is taken into the system, certain changes are noted in organs and tissues. Since all drugs are inert substances, whatever action is induced by their use is the result of a vital action of the body against them. It is the body that acts on the drug (not the other way around) and the drug is classified according to that action. For instance, certain drugs are termed cathartics or purgatives, which means that, when they are taken into the alimentary canal, they set up irritation in the bowel, and the result is that a copious amount of water is secreted there by the system so that the danger to the parts will be minimized. The final result is that the contents of the bowels are evacuated in order to get rid of the irritation, and the drug is said to have the power to move the bowels.

Then there are the diaphoretics and the diuretics—drugs which, when taken into the body, are quickly eliminated through the skin and the kidneys. If they were not eliminated in this way, they would set up changes in the tissues; therefore, all they do is to urge the system to get rid of them through the most appropriate channels. Such drugs have no power in themselves to add to the vital capacity of an organ. The living body is the actor—the drugs are acted upon.

It is because the chemical actions of these substances are destructive to the life of the cells that the body resists and expels them. It is the resistive and expulsive actions of the body that are commonly mistaken for the actions of drugs. Drugs are chemical substances and chemical action (union and disunion of elements) is the only kind of "action" of which they are capable. The actions of the body in resisting and expelling these substances are designed to prevent their chemical union with the constituents of the cells. The body seeks to preserve its integrity and to defend itself against injury. Its preservative and defensive actions are its own and not those of the drug.

More than a hundred years ago Hygienists defined poison. In medical literature there is only vagueness as to what constitutes a food, a poison, or a medicine.

Dr. Russell Thacker Trall, a hygienic pioneer, defined food: "Food includes all those substances whose elements are convertible into, and do form, the constituent matters of the tissues". The fact that stands out in this definition is that food is usable substance. It is something that the body can appropriate and make a part of itself. It is digested, absorbed, circulated, assimilated, and transformed into living structure. It should be obvious that any substance that cannot be so appropriated and transformed is not food. Whatever its relation to the living organism, it is not related to it as food.

What then is a poison? Again, we shall quote Trall: "Poisons are those articles or agencies which are not, in any form or quantity, convertible into any of the structures of the living body, nor employed by the organism in the performance of any of its functions". He went further in his definition and said: "Poisons are chemically incompatible with the functions of the living organism". This definition of Trall is incarnated in a hazy sort of way by the following definition from a medical dictionary: "A poison is any substance which, when ingested, inhaled, or absorbed, or when applied to, injected into or developed within the body, in relatively small amounts, by its chemical action may cause damage to structure or disturbance of function".

What we must understand is that:

1) "All drugs are chemically incompatible with the structures of the human body".

2) "All drugs are physiologically incompatible with the functions of the human body".

3) "All drugs are absolute poisons under all circumstances".

The evidence for these statements are the alleged modes of action of the drugs themselves. What phenomena indicate the so-called modus operandi of drugs? Pain, agitation, disorders of the body, derangement of the mind, nausea, vomiting, griping, spasms, trembling, dizziness, drunkenness, staggering, blindness, deafness, prostration, skin eruptions, ulcerations, blisters, paralysis, difficult breathing (asthma), rapid heart action, depressed heart action, and so on through a whole catalogue of abnormalities. Are these symptoms, signs, feelings, alterations of functions, effects, phenomena, operations or whatever you may prefer to call them, any part of the healthy or normal state of the body? If they are really abnormal, as Hygienists have contended from the very origin of the Hygienic movement, their causes are certainly incompatible with the normal or healthy state of the human body, hence functionally and physiologically incompatible. Drugs are not poisons in large doses, and medicines in small doses, but are always poisons. All the effects which follow their ingestion or injection, and which are mistakenly called medicinal, are themselves evidences of the destructive character of these chemicals.

The essence of toxicity is non-usability. The degree of toxicity of one drug, as compared to another, is somehow linked with the different degrees of incompatibility. That is to say that differences in the range of incompatibility measure the differences in virulence between different drugs. If a man swallows a drug, he is poisoned to a degree precisely proportionate to the quantity swallowed. It is the same whether he is well or sick, although the apparent effect would vary, both in kind and degree, according to the condition of his body at the time. But when he swallows at different times, two different drugs of the same dosage, the effects that follow will be determined by the degree of incompatibility of the two poisons.

What has emerged so far is the simple fact that when drugs are administered to the sick, be they in whatever form, e.g. alcohol, tea, coffee, tobacco, coca-cola, or prescribed by the physician, the result is disease. The diseases consequent upon the administration of drugs are so numerous and complicated, as we will see in later chapters, as to preclude the possibility of ever fully describing them. Thousands of patients, suffering with what were originally simple diseases, have been drugged into the worst complications conceivable. In nearly all, if not all such cases, Natural Hygiene care would have enabled these sufferers to return to full health in a brief time.

Dr. Oliver Wendell Holmes, Professor of Anatomy at Harvard University, used to say that "if all the drugs in the Pharmacopaeia were thrown into the sea, it would be good for humanity but bad for the fishes".

In the meantime, it is also good to see a physician writing in the British Medical Journal of January 25, 1969, under the caption: "Drug intervention in the common cold": "Perhaps we should look more closely at our patients' symptoms and consider them as outward manifestations of the continually changing factors which protect the body against infection. Our treatment might more profitably be directed at stimulating those processes which naturally overcome infection, rather than at killing off the bacteria or viruses which may be only one of many interacting factors in disease causation".

At the Conference of the Medical Association of New Zealand, another such warning was issued. The Auckland Star of March 1969 reported the Governor General, Sir Arthur Porritt, a famous surgeon, as saying that he "was shocked to read the New Zealand figures for prescription costs—a drug bill of more than 20 million dollars a year, plus six million on self-prescribed medicine". Then he posed the important question: "How little did the patient know of side-effects, and that use of drugs could limit the defenses and healing mechanisms of the body? How often did the doctor tell the patient of these things"? One wonders.

From time to time Hygienic and Nature Cure publications have quoted authorities to show that the one certain thing about drug therapy is that no one can be sure about its uncertainties.

The reaction of the patient may differ with age, with sex, and even with the time of the year, and there may even be variations in the same individual at different times of his life. We also learn that, according to a senior lecturer in the Department of Medicine, University of Liverpool, England, hereditary factors may dictate certain drug variations. The Medical News, December 15, 1967, quoted the doctor as saying: "It is quite wrong to regard unusual reactions to drugs as mere annoyances. In the future, dosage may need to be more personalized, and unusual toxic effects may be clues to more examples of inherited differences and may throw light on some chronic diseases".

⨍ In this respect a definition of drug adversity from the United States is worth recording: "What needs to be understood and incorporated into the modern definition of drug adversity is not the truism that most drugs or even all drugs are toxic (we have known this for a long time), but that all the effects of drugs—good, bad and indifferent —are examples of drug toxicity, a selective toxicity producing alterations in structure and function, *which by some happy chance are useful to the sick man, or by some misfortune make matters worse for him*". (Italics mine K.R.S.)

A. Albert, Selective Toxicity by Wiley, New York 1965

This then is medical science—and for the millionth time we ask those who perpetuate it: "Why then poison the sick?"

The pharmaceutical manufacturers are no exception to the rule that "Profits" are a powerful incentive in all forms of industry. In a supplement to the London Times, December 15, 1967, dealing with "The Pharmaceutical Industry Today", we find the following statement: "At least since the report of the 1959/60 Public Accounts Committee there has been a tendency to think that firms in the pharmaceutical industry make unduly high profits. On the bases of an examination of the accounts of 43 firms, the Public Accounts Committee found that the average rate of return on capital in the industry for the period 1955/59 was 26.7 percent, compared with an average of British Industry as a whole of about 16.7 percent, and that the eight most profitable companies retained a return of some 73 percent."

Pertaining to the same theme, there is yet another report from The Evening Star, Washington, D.C., October 25, 1967: "Three pharmaceutical companies, the biggest in the industry, have gone on trial in Manhattan Federal Court for conspiracy in alleged price-fixing of one billion dollars in broad spectrum antibiotics or so-called 'wonder drugs' ".

Many of you who read this believe, quite innocently, that the main purpose behind the use of drugs is the alleviation of disease, but there is another side of the question which cannot be ignored. The Manchester Guardian, December 19, 1967, reported that a Swedish lawyer is working on an investigation into the Thalidomide tragedy and quotes him as follows:

"I am trying to reveal how the pharmaceutical industry is working. It is the sacred cow of the chemical business. It doesn't sell goods like those you buy anywhere; they have an aura of something special. But the public must see that it is really like the iron industry or the clothing industry—it just wants to sell its products". And sell them they do; otherwise, there would be no need of a book like this one to expose the facts so few people are aware of.

According to a report in the New York Post, April 21, 1953, on the day President Eisenhower took office "one family in every five was in debt to its doctor in the U.S.A. The nation's total unpaid medical bill was estimated at $1,000,000,000." In Britain in 1953, according to the Minister of Health, "prescriptions were now running at the rate of 241 million a year, and the average cost of a prescription had climbed from 38 pence in 1949/50 to an estimated 52 pence for each prescription this year".

Many new medical treatments seem to go through the same pattern of development: At the first stage they are highly regarded and ofttimes widely publicized; then some doubts seem to creep in, and the procedure comes under some criticism; finally, warnings are issued of side-effects which had not been anticipated. New drugs are thus introduced at the rate of two per week and, because they have been tested on animals, it is assumed they are safe. Often they merely replace other drugs which have been in use long enough. In 1960, 113 new products were announced in The Pharmaceutical Index, and 48 were discontinued; in 1961, 81 new products were listed against 30 discontinued; and so it goes on.

The use of Hydrocortisone appears to have gone through such stages. "Warning on the Use of Hydrocortisone" ran a headline in the Medical News, June 21, 1968, which then reported as follows: "Hydrocortisone should not be injected directly into a joint more than once every month. This concensus was apparent after a paper presented to the Canadian Orthopaedic Association by a team from The Hospital for Sick Children. The paper was a follow-up which showed that when Hydrocortisone was used more often, it caused a lack of lustre, deceased cartilage thickness, calcific deposits, fissuring and fibrillation, cyst formation, necrosis and vascular invasion . . ."

This is a warning that no one can afford to ignore that drugs are poisons and do cause damage.

CHAPTER VI

The Effects of Drug Taking

"Gentlemen, ninety-nine out of every hundred medical facts are medical lies; and medical doctrines are, for the most part, stark, staring nonsense".

Prof. Gregory, M.D.

What is a Tonic? Medically speaking, it is a medicine that is said to invigorate—to strengthen and increase tone, as one medical dictionary puts it. God alone knows how many millions of tonics have been prescribed by medical practitioners over hundreds of years. If a drug or medicine had the power to "strengthen and increase tone" as simply as that, there should be a whole population of Herculean types walking around.

What is important to understand is that these medicines, like all others, are toxic to the body, and that it is only because of the selectivity of the system and its powers of elimination that great harm is not done. A good many physicians avoid prescribing but there are patients who have been so brainwashed by previous medical indoctrination that, especially after illness, if not during, they feel they must have a pick-me-up, so they insist on having their "tonics" and go on taking them for weeks afterwards.

They should be warned by a note from an article in Medical News, December 1966, written by an authority on pharmacology, which puts the "tonic" idea in perspective. The title of the article was "Science Disproves the 'Tonic' Fantasy" and the writer said, among other things, "This view of drugs as toxic agents is not shared by all members of the public, many of whom think of drugs as 'tonics', 'stimulants' or potent tissue foods. The scientific picture is at variance with this fantasy. Except in replacement therapy (a vitamin or hormone supplied in conditions of marked deficiency), the toxic nature of all drugs

70

makes it desirable to discontinue their use as early as possible".

This indeed is a death blow to all those who think that health can be obtained from a bottle and over a store counter. When will people learn that health is something to be worked for by effort and self-discipline in all walks of life and can only be achieved by those who have deserved it?

It is useless for the physicians to cry out that the public demands drugs. Who taught them to rely on such products for palliation of their systems? Who gave these people hope, with all the fanfare of a circus coming to town, that drugs will solve their ill-health problems? Who conditioned the public to believe and think that a sick body needs the administration of poisons to make it well? If now the physicians find that the tables have been turned and that their misdeeds of the past and present are there for all and sundry to see, then let them repent and make it their public duty to inform the people that they were wrong in letting them believe that drugs can make a sick person well and a well person even better.

If treatment turns one form of disease into two, it is difficult to see what purpose it serves. For example, in the newsletter of the Arthritis & Rheumatism Council for Research, 1967, we are told that a grant has been made for research into the effects of some common drugs on the kidneys of some people. It says, "Aspirin, phenacitin, and other drugs are invaluable for the relief of pain, which is the most unpleasant feature of arthritis. These drugs have been used with apparent safety for many years, but it has been found that a small proportion of people who regularly take them, develop serious kidney disease". The operative words here are, of course, "apparent safety" because for many years these drugs were wrongly thought to be harmless, whereas they were in fact disease-producing. In short, arthritis plus drugging produces other diseases.

Let us keep in mind the following quotation from a book review in the Medical News, July 2, 1965: "All drugs are potentially toxic, and so the crucial question about a drug is not whether it is toxic but how toxic it is and what factors modify this toxicity". All we need to remember is that "toxic" and "toxicity" are euphemisms for poisonous and poison-potency and that, while it is true that certain factors may modify the toxicity of the drugs, other factors may also increase it. Fresh evidence is constantly coming to light which shows that alcohol and drug combination may make drug-taking more perilous, and even certain foods—like cheese, can alter adversely drug reactions.

In Nature, July 6, 1968, there was a report from the divisions of Allergy, Immunology and Rheumatology, Scripps Clinic and Foundation, La Jolla, California, in which further effects of aspirin were described. It said, " 'Aspirin Intolerance', a syndrome characterized by asthma, rhinitis, and nasal polyps, has been recognised for some years and is induced by the ingestion of aspirin". It went on, "Numerous other reactions such as abnormal renal function in rheumatoid arthritis, analgesis nephropathy, massive gastric haemorrhage, abnormal haemostasis caused by hypoprothrombinaemia and impaired platelet function, pancytopenia, and encephalopathy have been ascribed to the ingestion of aspirin".

In simple words, it means that the taking of aspirin causes adverse reactions in the kidneys, the intestines, the blood, and the brain. What is of interest to us is that aspirin has been in common use for nearly a century, and yet the researchers are still discovering new and unexpected reactions induced by this common household remedy. This should be an object lesson to us all. For many years the same self-styled authorities assured us that aspirin was a safe and simple pain killer, and now the tune is changing. In view of this, we must ask ourselves what value we can place on the assurances of medical scientists about various other drugs, about fluoridation, artificial sweeteners, pesticides, and chemicals and colourings in our foods, about demineralized, devitalised, denatured, foodless foods like white sugar, white flour, and a host of other things. The fact is that, as with aspirin, no one can predict what the long-term effect will be until the experiment has been made, and then the damage may have been done.

The Sunday Times of January 15, 1967 put this very succinctly: "Most patients assume that when their doctor prescribes a drug, he knows about it. The chances are he knows very little about it. Half the drugs now being used were not on the market five years ago. With this rate of innovational advance, a doctor is out of date five years after qualification".

Because no one can predict just what effect a drug will produce in the body, the most careful of physicians must still be regarded as experimenters. This point is brought out in a case in the United States where it was found that a woman was given a drug for arthritis which "caused a degeneration of cells in the retina of the eyes that resulted in an 80 percent loss of vision". The Washington Post of March 17, 1969, reporting on the case, said that "drugs potent enough to injure and kill are often prescribed casually and even carelessly because of excessive reliance by the medical profession on detailmen, as the salesmen are usually referred to". It makes one wonder where all the so-called scientific training of a physician comes in if he is to be given his lessons by a salesman of vested interests.

No doubt the physicians at the British Medical Association Meeting in 1962 were forced to admit that "we are moving from the age of dangerous surgery into the age of dangerous medicine".

As we have shown in the first chapter, drugs promising marvellous cures fail to deliver the goods. "Wonder drugs" often emerge as "Blunder drugs".

In 1948 Professor Philip Hench of the Mayo Clinic, U.S.A., discovered cortisone as a cure for rheumatism. With great ballyhoo it was praised sky high. But recently, when a committee set up by the Medical Research Council and the Nuffield Foundation examined all the claims, they found that in early and uncomplicated rheumatoid arthritis, cortisone was no more effective than aspirin. Then a new wonder drug called pregnenolone, known as "the poor man's cortisone" was produced but, after another brief interlude, it was declared "not promising for use against arthritis" by the National Arthritis & Rheumatism Foundation (U.S.A.).

In 1952 Lord Horder, speaking to the British Rheumatic Foundation, issued the following warning: "It is a mistaken idea that as a result of taking these cortisone and allied remedies, patients with rheumatoid arthritis are cured. This is not true. Cortisone is giving us more rheumatic patients left at the stage where their disabilities require treatment than before they took cortisone".

In 1960, at the height of the cholesterol scare, an American drug called MER/29 was put on the market with powerful medical backing. MER/29, it was claimed, was going to solve the cholesterol problem. But in October, 1962 it was admitted that MER/29 had side-effects causing cataract of the eye, peeling skin, impotence, and unpleasant effects on the reproductive organs. In April, 1963 the drug was withdrawn.

A similar thing occurred with a drug Banthine, discovered in 1949, a complex ammonium compound which would paralyse gastric nerve action, block the impulses of the vagus nerves, and thus control the secretion of acid and digestive juices. It was mailed as the saviour of sufferers from gastric and duodenal ulcers. Soon, however, it was discovered that this wonder drug had blundered like so many others, causing checked gastric secretions, acting on salivary glands and drying up the mouth, dilating the pupils of the eyes, giving some double vision, and, because it relaxed the stomach muscles, causing constipation in others. Soon it too disappeared from the news.

Another drug, Librium, used for emotional and mental disorders, was described as "the greatest boon to mind doctors". Then it was discovered that its after-effects included drowsiness, with loss of capacity to think clearly, giddiness, and states of confusion with spells of fainting without warning, and increased appetite and increased weight gain. Another drug as commonly prescribed as librium for mental and emotional disorders is Valium. Valium is known to cause a fairly wide range of side-effects, including drowsiness, lightheadedness, loss of control over movements of arms, legs, etc., low blood pressure, headaches, blurred vision, nausea, impaired memory, slurred speech, skin rash, incontinence and constipation.

These drug failures and a thousand more have not yet taught the medical profession that drugs never cure—that they can only alleviate pain at best and make life bearable while the body repairs and restores itself, and that recovery can be accelerated by fasting, rest, correct diet, deep breathing and fresh air, exercise and emotional poise.

Sir Derek Dunlop (Emeritus Professor of Therapeutic Medicine at Edinburgh and Chairman of the Ministry of Health Committee on Safety of Drugs), summed up in a few sentences the predicament of the modern-day physician in a lecture he gave under the auspices of the British Medical Association at Cardiff, Wales, in 1965.

"At his best", he said, "the Victorian doctor did more good, and certainly less harm, than the worst of the moderns, who would prescribe a bottle of sulpha tablets for a sick child, then try some injections of penicillin, and, if that were unavailing, tetracycline pills. Then, with the situation hopelessly confused, he would not have the faintest idea whether the continuing fever was due to the persistence of the disease process or to the effects of his own medicaments". There can be no more telling comment than this in this whole story of the blind leading the blind.

We Hygienists contend that acute symptoms of disease are a kind of warning and the body's own attempt to cleanse and purify itself of the toxic load in the system which, on reaching a certain point of accumulation, leads to toxaemia. For example, a fever, cold, cough, diarrhoea, skin eruptions and so on are life-saving attempts by the body towards decongestion. Stopping the body in its effort towards such self-purification measures leads not only to prolongation of acute distress symptoms, but gradually brings about chronic changes in the structure and functions of the tissues involved. The taking of drugs hinders and interferes with this life-saving effort. The effects of drug-taking are not remedial but disease-producing.

Asthma is said to be an allergic disease affecting perhaps half a million people in Britain. It has been with us for a very long time and so there have been plenty of opportunities for its study and for the application of almost every imaginable treatment. Yet, according to published statements, medicine has made no progress—indeed, it seems to have regressed. Two items regarding asthma appeared in the Medical Journal of Australia, May 10, 1969: "Death from Asthma in the 19th century was considered very rare by the outstanding physicians of that time. According to the United States Public Health Service vital statistics, however, the sharp rise came between 1930 and 1953, when it rose from less than 30, up until 1930 to a peak of 6,737 in 1953 . . ."

The other statement came from the book *Bedside Medicine* by Dr. Snapper, published in 1967, which seemed to confirm the above observation: "Between 1886 and 1906, when autopsies could be obtained more easily than nowadays, only seven autopsy cases of status asthmaticus were published. Evidently hardly ever did anybody die of an asthmatic attack. The fact that nowadays nearly every hospital pathology museum includes several cases of status asthmaticus illustrates that the addition of tranquillizers, barbiturates, etc., has strongly potentiated the dangers of this allergic condition".

Apparently the joke about "Doctor, what should I do, I have a shocking cold?" "Go out into the cold with a minimum of clothing and get thoroughly soaked in the rain", replied the physician. "But I am sure to get pneumonia, Doctor", said the patient. "Never mind that—we can cure pneumonia with a shot of penicillin—but we can't do a damn thing with your cold", replied the doctor, is applicable to asthma and a host of other diseases.

For years Hygienists have warned people against taking aspirin for colds, in spite of the doctor's routine prescription of two aspirins and rest in bed. Such a warning was said by many to be just cranky. But many doctors are coming around to the Hygienist viewpoint, and yet another protest against this practice is given in the London Sunday Times of July 13, 1969, which printed the opinion of Dr. Avery Jones, who is a physician to the Department of Gastroenterology at the Central Middlesex Hospital. The report said: "Dr. Jones warned that aspirin should not be taken for colds and simple respiratory infections because even small amounts can cause minor bleeding from the stomach and gut in 80 percent of people. *Medium doses can upset the stomach, especially in cases of colds;* larger amounts of the drug occasionally produce dangerous haemorrhage. One patient in his wards had to have 14 pints of blood transfused after taking four aspirin tablets four times a day for the common cold", (Italics mine K.R.S.)

If ever there was a case in which the remedy is more dangerous than the ailment, this is surely it. Far better when you have a cold is to abstain from all food except water, i.e. Fast and go to bed, and rest and keep warm. At least you won't have any such repercussion as gastric haemorrhage.

If medicine were an exact science, then results could be predicted; if we regard it as an art, one accepts the fact that the methods are empirical and the results unpredictable. Drug therapy, at best, is not a science and never was, but an art, as is admitted by many authorities. For instance, in an article in the London Evening Standard, February 10, 1967, headed "The World of Science looks at the Drug Industry", we get some idea of how little is known of why drugs behave as they do when taken in the body. The article goes on to say: "In the never-ending war against disease, the men who seek, discover, and produce drugs have come up with some formidable weapons in their time . . . The hunt for new drugs goes on. But the discovery rate is slackening—primarily because all the obvious substances have been looked at at least once. So Britain's pharmaceutical industry is adjusting its research effort to place more emphasis on learning how existing drugs work in the body. In particular, it is looking at what is happening inside the cell . . ."

If it is not known how drugs work in the body or what effect they may have inside the cells, how is it possible to use such an agent in a rational manner? When will they learn that all so-called actions of drugs "therapeutic and physiological", are actions of the body in an attempt at prompt removal of the same? Drugs put in a dead body produce no outward manifestation of such actions because the living body with life in it as the actor, is dead.

In all the publicity that is at the present time being given to the tragic subject of drug addiction, very little has been said about the danger of drugs used for so-called therapeutic purposes and the need for abolition of all such drugs. Indeed, we can say with truth that it is only in Hygienic and nature-cure circles that this point has been emphasized. It is gratifying, therefore, to see a prominent surgeon giving some attention to this matter. In the London Times of March 3, 1967 he discussed addiction and publicity and calls attention to "the present dangers of all forms of drug-taking, even those for therapeutic purposes . . . it would be wonderful if the press, police, and public could combine in wiping out the dangers of the present epidemic. This involves not only legislation and punitive action but means restraint in the use and control of all therapeutic drugs as well as those of addiction".

With respect, we would urge him to give this advice to his own profession—the physicians and surgeons. The public only do what they are conditioned to do by those supposed to be in authority. The same paper reported "some barbiturate drugs, taken during pregnancy, could sometimes produce a depression of the child's respiratory centre when it was born, so that it did not take its first breath".

We ask the medical profession, the public, and all those who perpetuate the drug industry—is human life not sacred enough, that it should be sacrificed in your blind pursuit of obstinate and obsolete principles? Before more human lives and other living organisms are maimed or destroyed by wholesale drug therapy all over the world, the truth about the effects of drug taking must be made known, and the sooner the better.

An extract from the Journal of the American Medical Association should frighten all sensible people who are willing to know more about the effects of drug taking. Here it is: "These toxic effects include gastro-intestinal bleeding from salicylates (aspirin), renal papillary necrosis from phenylbutazone, dermatitis and renal complications from gold salts, retinal damage from antimalarials, purpura, peptic ulcer and osteoporosis from cortico steroids and gastro-intestinal and cerebral complications from the use of indomethacin".

CHAPTER VII

Some Drug—Induced Diseases
(Iatrogenic)

"In their zeal to do good, physicians have done much harm. They have hurried many to the grave, who would have recovered if left to nature".

Prof. Alonzo Clark, M.D.

The idea that we shall be able to conquer diseases by drug-therapy has been proven fallacious, since drugs in themselves are causative of disease. Some figures from the United States show that something like ten percent of hospitalized cases are drug-induced, and a recent study indicated that one case out of every seven in hospitals for gastro-intestinal bleeding was due to aspirin. This figure was given by Drs. Max and Menguy of the University of Chicago, and it was cited by them at the clinical congress of the American College of Surgeons.

Research done by these doctors showed that aspirin prevented the formation of the natural protective mucus of the intestinal walls and prevented the surface cells from renewing themselves. In its report of this investigation, Osteopathic News, November/December, 1968, said: "The enormity of the problem was cited by Drs. Max and Menguy, who noted that more than 20 million pounds of aspirin are consumed each year, and aspirin is responsible for one out of every seven patients hospitalized for gastro-intestinal bleeding".

When we bear in mind that this may be the result of using what for so long has been considered to be a safe household remedy, we get some idea of what the more powerful drugs may do to the body, and we need not be surprised that already four volumes, some of which we will quote, have been published dealing with "drug-induced diseases", which makes the idea of conquering disease by drug therapy a hollow one indeed.

Here is an item which needs no comment. "In Beverly Hills, California, 'flu' victim actress, Joan Tabor, 34-year-old former wife of actor Broderick Crawford, died after mistakenly taking too much of the prescribed medicine..." *Excerpt from the London Evening Standard, December 19, 1968.*

About 150 years ago Dr. Sylvester Graham, a pioneer of Natural Hygiene, warned people about the use of table salt: "From my own extended and careful observations during the last eight years, I have been strongly pressed to the conclusion that dietetic use of salt is largely concerned in the production of cancers and other glandular diseases of the human system, and I am certain that it aggravates many chronic diseases". Many people do not realize that salt is a drug and a poison. However, even the medical profession is beginning to realize that it can well be so. According to the science report in the London Times, September 30, 1968, it may now be thinking again about the subject. The report went on: "New evidence supporting an earlier proposal that the level of blood pressure is related to the intake of dietary salt is set out in an article in the September issue of the "New England Journal of Medicine . . ." The evidence came from a study of people living in the Northern Cook Islands, whose habits differed, especially in relation to their salt intake. The conclusion seemed to support the hypothesis that salt does affect blood pressure".

In January 1976 the papers reported that doctors were worried about salt being added to the National Dried Milk, as they believed it was instrumental in causing the deaths in young babies described as "cot-deaths".

A report published in the Santa Barbara News Press, U.S.A., June 29, 1967, gives some idea of the way in which drugs used for so-called "therapeutic" means turn a killer. It concerned the report made by Dr. L. E. Cluff, professor of medicine at the University of Florida, to a sub-committee. Dr. Cluff claimed that his findings were backed by a six-year study. "Adverse effects of non-prescription drugs, as well as prescription ones, are responsible for hospitalization and death of a significant number of patients". Some of his figures about the adverse effects of drugs gives one an idea of the magnitude of the problem: "Four to five percent of patients admitted for hospital medical service are found to have adverse drug reactions, while three to four percent are admitted because of drug illness. Ten percent experience ill effects from drugs, while hospitalized. Twenty percent of adverse reactions are caused by non-prescription drugs such as laxatives, analgesics, and antacids. Eighty percent are caused by such prescription items as penicillin, digitalis, sedatives, and tranquillizers. Drug illness involving medical service was the seventh most common cause of hospitalization. In one three-month study, 36 to 714 patients were admitted with drug illness; eight died. Of 67 becoming ill because of drugs while in hospital, three died". Dear reader, you have been warned.

Children suffered for many years from a peculiar disease which baffled medical diagnosticians. It was known as "pink disease" and was said to be of unknown origin. It was characterised by mental, nutritional and skin disorders, there being intense itching of the hands and feet, while the skin was subject to various rashes, together with changes in its colour, ranging from pink to brown. The mucous membranes of the body were also adversely affected, especially those of the mouth, where ulcers sometimes formed. The teeth softened, and there were changes in the digestive system and in the function of the kidneys, which were so severe that in some cases the child did not survive the disease. Finally, someone observed that these symptoms resembled those of mercurial poisoning, and the problem of the disease was then well on the way to a solution. Eventually the trouble was found to be due to a drug called Calomel—a mercurial preparation which was used in the teething powders which were given freely to infants in those times.

Another example of such gross negligence on the part of the medical profession is to be found in a small booklet called "Do Medicines Cause Disease", by James C. Thomson, the great pioneer of Nature Cure in Great Britain, and published in 1942. In it he writes: "Do you, Mr. Brown, realize that one of the most carefully guarded secrets of the medical profession is the great physiological destruction wrought in patients' tissues through the medicines called "alternatives"—mercury, iodine, and arsenic? Although the public does not know it, that is why they are afraid of syphilis. The dreadful "later stages" are exclusively due to the medicaments used in the treatment of earlier symptoms. All accepted authorities deliberately confuse the issue in such matters, e.g. Professor Clark in Applied Pharmacology, admits: "It is difficult, if not impossible, to decide the relative responsibility of the drug and of the pathological lesions"—which is as near as an orthodox authority could go towards confessing that the later symptoms of "the disease" are due to alternative poisoning. All orthodox teachers are at great pains to ignore the shattering experiments of Dr. Hermann of Vienna, who proved beyond a shadow of doubt that syphilis under hygienic living is self-limited and, treated without alternatives, develops no further symptoms.

For thirty years Dr. Hermann was Superintendent of the Venereal Wards in the Hospital Weiden, near Vienna, one of the greatest institutions in the world for the treatment of syphilis and allied ailments. He treated sixty thousand cases of venereal disease without the use of mercury. In no single case thus treated and cured did he have a record of spontaneous recurrence, of the alleged tertiary symptoms or hereditary transmission".

Do we need to ask the question, "Do medicines cause disease?"

Let us now take Phenacetin, a drug which for many years has been extensively used in self-medication and widely advertised as a household remedy. Warnings have come from many sources, and the Manchester Guardian, August 3, 1968, had this headline: "Warning of Drug Danger". The paper reported that "Mr. F. Hails, the Stoke-on-Trent coroner, said yesterday that a woman had died after being 'trapped' by tablets containing the drug Phenacetin". The woman died from kidney failure. An article in the British Medical Journal, March 13, 1965, said "Phenacetin has been used continuously in treatment for almost 80 years and is contained in many proprietary preparations . . . The association of Phenacetin with renal damage was not described until the 1950s, and the reports emphasized several features common to the cases . . . clinically these patients usually presented with features of acute or chronic renal failure, and at necropsy the kidneys might be normal or reduced in size, and showed papillary necrosis". All of which goes to prove that no drug is safe, in spite of long usage and medical approval. (A drug does not change its nature because it has been prescribed to you by a medical physician. It remains a poison under all circumstances.)

Treating the symptoms of disease instead of eradicating causative factors in our habits of day to day living is likely to provide the wrong answer almost every time. This has been proven in the treatment of peptic ulcers, when the prescribed diets and medicines have sometimes produced scurvy, among other troubles. Now, a report comes from the U.S.A., which suggests that the milk and antacids which are so often used in these cases may make matters worse: "Milk and antacids, the mainstays of therapy for peptic ulcers, may lead to metabolic alterations potentially more serious than the primary disease being treated, Donald Berkowitz, M.D. warned recently".

The doctor went on to say that such treatment might produce many changes in the system, including the development of gout. Naming this as a new disease pattern in itself—the milk-alkali syndrome—he called upon the profession to realize "the necessity of re-evaluating and reappraising these therapeutic concepts in the light of newer findings and beliefs, with the hope that these undesirable side-effects of the medical treatment of peptic ulcer be prevented". His explanation of the trouble was that this treatment upset the acid-alkaline balance in the system and led to alkalosis if long continued.

Let us take another drug, Butazolidine, so commonly used for rheumatism. Toxic reactions occur in some 25 to 40 percent of patients taking Butazolidine, and they are often sufficiently severe to cause the withdrawal of the drug. They appear to arise less frequently in men than in women. Most common reactions are nausea, rash; vertigo, oedema (fluid retention), mouth inflammation, blurred vision, insomnia, epigastric pain, and diarrhoea. More severe reactions include reactivation of gastric and duodenal ulcers, with perforation, vomiting of blood, melaenia (blood in stools), hepatitis, hypertension and, more rarely, agranulocytosis, thrombocytopaenia, and aplastic anaemia. Yet a report from the United States makes it look as though all the drugs given for rheumatism and arthritis are making no headway at all in easing the progress of the diseases concerned. "Figures obtained in 1966/67 by the U.S.

Public Health Service and released by the Arthritis Foundation show that 16.8 million people in the United States, (one out of every 11), are suffering from some form of arthritis. The old figure was one in 16. This is an increase of more than 3 million over previous estimates of the country's arthritic population. Approximately 3.4 million arthritis patients are disabled at any one time, and the annual cost to the national economy—including annual wage losses and medical care costs—is estimated at more than 3.5 billion dollars".

As we have said before, no part of the body escapes the harm done to it by taking one or other kind of drugs. Many rashes and skin complaints are eliminative actions of the body, and they may have many different causes. It is well known that they are not unusual accompaniments of drug-therapy. The Practitioner, January 1969 issue, reported: "Unexplained rashes, possibly due to drugs, are a recurring problem in practice. Unfortunately, few of these rashes are diagnostic of any particular drug, and one drug may produce eruptions of varying morphology in different individuals. Antibiotics as a group seem to be the commonest cause of drug rashes and of the antibiotics ampicillin is the most frequent offender".

The same journal also reported: "Iatrogenic dermatoses (those due to treatment) are of common occurrence and, with the introduction of more and more powerful drugs, will become increasingly common. A report from the Johns Hopkins Hospital indicated that four percent of admissions were due to such adverse reactions . . ."

None of their boasted claims have ever materialised for the drug-pushers in the long run. Many people are under the impression that pneumonia is one of the diseases which modern drug therapy has conquered, and so it must have come as something of a shock to them to read in the London Sunday Times, January 19, 1969, that "more than 32,000 people died from the pneumonias in England and Wales in 1967 (and 36,000 in 1966) but there is no reliable estimate of how many were due to Pneumococci. If the U.S. vaccine gives protection, the Medical Research Council will probably decide to have some kind of pneumonia vaccine developed and tested in Britain for offer to high risk groups—notably victims of the English disease, chronic bronchitis". Dr. Edwin Lerner, the co-ordinator of the research programme in that country, said that the vaccine idea was withdrawn in 1952 because, as he put it, "Penicillin was the cure-all in those days, and we thought we could cure them".

But way back in 1953 Dr. W. A. Altemeier, Chairman of the Department of Surgery at the University of Cincinnati School of Medicine, said, "Pencillin is much less effective than when it was introduced ten years ago".

The antibiotics, it seems, have had their day. Take, for instance, the use of the drug chloromycetin. It was first marketed in 1949 and, because it was then thought to be harmless, it was prescribed to millions of people—and we mean literally millions, especially in the United States. In that country in 1960, the sales of the drug reached 86 million dollars. In the Medical News, April 5, 1968, we read that "American doctors will receive personal appeals from the Government to heed stricter warnings to be issued against the misuse of the antibiotic, chloromycetin. Excess prescribing of the drug has been linked with an alarming number of deaths and grave illnesses stemming from blood disorders. Witnesses testifying at the U.S. Senate Small Business Monopoly Sub-Committee said that most of the 70 million dollars worth of chloromycetin sold each year was used for colds, acne, and other minor ailments against the regulations of the Food & Drug Administration." The reason for limiting the use of this drug ought surely to frighten people: "A new label on the drug would warn that leukemia was a possible side-effect . . . the antibiotic was also said to cause aplastic anaemia . . ."

Another antibiotic which made headlines one way or another is Ceporin. The London Sunday Times, January 24, 1965, carried this headline, "New Drug 'Not Such a Miracle'". It went on: "The Consumers' Association confirmed on Friday that Glaxo's recent antibiotic, Ceporin, which was hailed by the lay press as Britain's new miracle drug, is considerably less miraculous than the nation's doctors and newspapers believed".

The report went on to tell of side-effects: "In patients already treated with the drug so far, a few have developed rashes and drug fever, suggesting that sensitization to it may occur fairly readily".

In the opinion of Kern and Wimberley (quoted by Leo Schindel, M.D., in his "Unexpected Reactions to Modern

Therapeutics," page 16): "Pencillin today heads the list of drugs which cause most frequently and most severely various hypersensitivity reactions . . . exceeds by far the heterogen serum reactions which often cause fatal shock and is responsible today for the increasing number of fatalities brought about by irreversible vascular allergies . . ."

"It is estimated that up to 1957 about one thousand fatal reactions to penicillin treatment had occurred in the United States alone . . ." (Press release, World Health Organisation—WHO-58, quoted by L. Meyler, M.D. in "Side Effects of Drugs"—1960, page 99).

As for Streptomycin, Leo Schindel, M.D., in his book, "Unexpected Reactions to Modern Therapeutics," page 37, says: "In respect to side-effects and toxicity, Streptomycin occupies a special position among antibiotics. There is hardly a side-effect accompanying the use of other antibiotics which has not been observed with Streptomycin".

". . . Intrathecal (intraspinal) injection can result in such severe side-effects as shock-like conditions with irregular breathing of reduced tempo, apnoea, fever, cramps and eventually, death. In the series of 90 cases presented by McKay, 14 cases of the above symptoms are recorded. Five of these latter died, probably as a result of the streptomycin therapy". (Ibid. page 47)

Coming back to Chloromycetin, we find that it is "A chloramphenical derivative for treatment of infections. Undesirable side-effects include masculinization. Others in the chloramphenicol family are now briefly described: chloramphenicol—used in cases of otitis caused necrotizing inflammation of the pharynx, soft palate and mucous membranes of the mouth and tongue.

Extended use leads to lowered resistance to candida organisms. Cases are recorded in which multiple abscesses of the brain have been formed; micro-abscesses in the heart, lungs, adrenals and kidneys; perforation of the duodenum; paralysis of the legs and lower part of the body; blood disorders including aplastic anaemia and granulocytosis; fatal thrombocytopenic purpura; and sciatic nerve injury. Leo Schindel, M.D. ("Unexpected Reactions" page 72) concludes that: "The fatalities accompanying chloramphenicol therapy, especially the occurrence of fatal aplastic anaemias, have at times sharply limited the use of this antibiotic".

From the book, "The Medicated Society", by Samuel Proger, M.D., we read this, "From a single antibiotic in 1942 we now have available at least 37 such drugs for human use, and this number will undoubtedly increase over the years. The quantity of these compounds produced in the United States for medical purposes is staggering. Information furnished by the chemical division of the U.S. Tariff Commission indicates that 455,000 pounds of penicillin were manufactured in 1955, 859,000 pounds in 1960 and 1961 ... In 1960, 287,000 pounds of tetracycline compounds were produced; in 1965, this rose to 2,544,750 pounds . . . the total quantities of all antibiotics made for human use in 1955 was 79,000,000 pounds; in 1960, 114,-000,000 pounds and in 1965 162,000,000 pounds".

With these figures in mind, we can ask whether these diseases, for which antibiotics are used, increase in proportion to the production of the drugs; surely with such miracle drugs one should expect a decrease in their use year by year. But, as the author goes on to say, "The antibiotics coin is not all glitter. It also has its dark side. All of these drugs have the capacity for harm. The frequency and severity of the reactions they produce vary with each compound, and to some extent with the person treated. All antibiotics produce allergic responses. Some of these are mild, but others are very severe and may even be fatal; for example, death has followed a single injection of penicillin in persons sensitized to this substance. Various kinds of skin rashes may develop during the use of these agents. Some are inherently toxic and damage the ears, kidneys, liver, and blood. A few cause vomiting and diarrhoea when taken by mouth. All, when given in conventional doses, alter the numbers and types of bacteria normally present in the nose, throat and lower intestinal tract. Most people suffer no ill-effects from such changes; a few are infected by their own bacteria. In these instances, the drug, while curing one infection, provokes the development of another, which may be more severe and life-threatening than the one for which treatment was initially given".

Can you believe that information of this type is daily coming out into the open, that the medical profession are aware of it but are doing nothing positive to stop the use of drugs? How can they believe, apart from being self-hypnotized, that drugs do help, when all evidence shows that they do nothing of the kind?

Perhaps a quotation by Panel Moderator. Dr. W. B. Carson, of Potsdam, New York, in the Medical News, May 14, 1965, should be hung up in the surgeries and consulting rooms of all physicians everywhere. Here it is: "I, personally, don't mind doctors acting like God. What I object to is their believing it themselves". Giving most of them the benefit of the doubt, may I add that when they stop believing in their omnipotent knowledge, they will then have the grace to stop acting as if human lives were some toys to be played about with.

On this very subject in January/February, 1976, Professor Peter Huntingford of London Hospital, when interviewed on B.B.C. Television said: "I think the time has come to question every piece of medical knowledge, every piece of medical advice that is given, and that patients should be able to say 'I don't believe what you are saying', or, 'I don't like the way you are doing it. Are there any choices? Why can't I be involved in the choice?'" This is startling advice from a medical professor and must be welcomed and acted upon by the public in general.

It would be useful to give a full list of all the drugs ever employed by the medical profession showing how each in turn had some deleterious effect on the living body, but that would involve writing volumes. However, we wish to mention a few selected at random.

Thalidomide—There is no need to belabour the point concerning this, as its disastrous effects are with us in the shape of deformed children to act as a constant reminder, but it should not be thought that only that one drug, marketed under the name of Distaval, was implicated.

Aminopterin—An agent used to induce abortion—usually ineffective—may cause malformation of the skull when the baby is born.

Androgens and Progestogens—These sex hormones sometimes used in endocrine and gynaecological disorders can cause masculinization of the female foetus.

Iodides and Thiourea—These treatments may cause congenital goitre.

Stelazine—Marketed under the name of Trifluperazine. It is recommended for a number of conditions, including "nausea and vomiting associated with pregnancy", but a communication from Canada to The Medical News, January 11, 1963 (page 10), warns that it is suspected of causing cases of congenital deformities. Eight such cases are mentioned in which this drug was taken by the mother during pregnancy. Other brand names under which this drug is marketed are: Parstelin, Stelabid, and Parstelin S12.

Asmaval—Prescribed for the prevention of asthmatic attacks and relief of congestion in hay fever, etc., contains one-fifth of a grain of Thalidomide in each tablet, and the recommended dosage is one or two tablets thrice daily, representing a daily intake of between three-fifths and one and one-fifth grains of Thalidomide.

Phenothiazine—Tranquillizer, causes undoubted retinal damage to the eyes.

Thloroquine—As above.

Meprobomate—Prescribed as a tranquillizing drug. Potentially toxic . . . Reports concerning 6,500 patients so treated include 23 attempted suicides and 113 anaphylactoid reactions including gastro-intestinal symptoms, blurred vision, impotence, menstrual irregularities. Also implicated as being possibly teratogenic (caused deformed babies).

Aminophylline—Another stimulant (pep pill) has listed as its poisoning effects anxiety, restlessness, agitation, vomiting, delirium, haematemesis, convulsions, coma, disturbed vision, confusion, paralysis of respiration, dehydration, shock, death.

In addition to all those listed above, there were some 2,400 drugs listed in a compilation prepared by L. Meyler, M.D., of "Unwanted Effects of Drugs" as reported in the Medical Literature of the World during the period 1958/1960.

A further edition of this publication which appeared in 1963 contained an additional 50 percent of new material, and more in a subsequent edition in the 1970s.

All these had been submitted to exhaustive tests on live animals and such tests failed to reveal (as was inevitable) the hidden dangers for human beings.

The following quotation from a recent publication "The Medicated Society" by Samuel Proger, M.D., exemplifies this difficulty: "Chlorothiazide is an example. This diuretic eliminates sodium, to be sure, but physicians immediately noticed that it also caused the loss of sodium's sister element, potassium. Depletion of the body's potassium is always undesirable and sometimes can produce damaging effects, especially on the kidneys. The answer was to give potassium supplements to the patient along with the diuretic. A more serious side-effect of the thiazides was not observable for many months after the diuretics went into general use. Then physicians noticed that gout and diabetes were appearing in patients who had been free of either disease. In fact, even the drugs used to prevent complications may themselves cause difficulties. Hence, the potassium supplements given in enteric-coated tablets, for the purpose of replacing potassium loss, were found many months later to cause occasional intestinal ulceration and obstruction. The moral of the tale is that the long-term use of any new drug may produce late, and unexpected, harmful effects. Before a physician can be entirely certain that a drug is doing more good than harm, he must cautiously observe for years the effects of a drug".

So let us re-examine the case for taking into our bodies drugs—no matter in what form—whether they be present in an article of diet, since chemicalization of foods is fast taking place, or are prescribed by a physician for major or minor ills. Let us ponder and reflect when we read such items as written in the "Medical News," April 19, 1968: "About 100 drug-induced deaths have been reported in England each year, since 1964, and some two-fifths of the fatalities were caused almost equally by two groupings of drugs—analgesics, antiarthritics and tranquillizer-depressants . . . Among the first group, phenylbutazone, an antiarthritic drug, seemed to be the cause of most deaths, Dr. Wills told the joint meeting of the American College of Physicians and the Royal College of Physicians of London". And here, just for the record, is an account of the effects of a new hypnotic-drug potentiation, taken from the same journal: "The effects were nosebleeding (6), dryness of mouth (10), swelling of tongue (4), tongue dry, furred, with brownish discoloration and fissuring (10 in varying degree), dryness of the lips and cracking of angles of mouth (5), dizziness and disorientation (7), and menstrual disturbances (2)".

Let us remind ourselves, like the writer in the Evening Star, Washington D.C., February 15, 1968, that ". . . American history reveals that the most significant decline in our death rate took place before the advent of vaccines and antibiotics, and that the dramatic difference they made was in large measure due to the already favourable environment on which they were superimposed. By the time there were vaccines for the prevention of polio and measles, most children were well enough nourished to permit their systems to respond with high levels of protective antibodies. By the time there were antibiotics, sanitation was good enough to make reinfection with other germs unlikely . . ."

If anyone wants further proof of the validity of such facts, they should look to those parts of the world where there is still malnourishment and a lack of sanitation. Appropriate to the above, we real in the London Times, February 25, 1966, an important article on the drug treatment of malaria; it concluded with this significant paragraph: "Finally—but by no means least—comes an intensification of the World Health Organisation campaign for the eradication of malaria. Drugs can never be more than a temporary expedient. The logical goal is the eradication of disease".

To conclude this chapter, I want to quote from an article in the Medical News, April 18, 1969, reporting on a B.M.A. clinical meeting in Malta. It carried the headline, "The Increasing Problems of Iatrogenic Disease", and said: "Opening a session devoted to iatrogenic diseases, Professor Ronald H. Girdwood, of Edinburgh, recalled that in a survey of patients in the medical wards of Johns Hopkins Hospital in the U.S.A. in 1966, no less than five percent were admitted on account of drug reaction; 3.9 percent had such an event as a contributory factor to admission and 13.6 percent had drug reactions during their stay in hospital".

The full circle has been reached—man in his false attempts to dominate nature in the field of biology has had to admit defeat. He has had to admit defeat and retreat when nature started hitting back. Man must learn to cooperate with nature and live a life where he fulfills the requisitions of Life and Living, whether it be in the spheres of diet and nutrition, rest and sleep and relaxation, vigorous activity and exercise, fresh air and sunshine, emotional poise and physiological rest, and his attitude towards the world and his environment. Unless man learns to fulfill these conditions of life, life will be denied to him, and he will only know disease, suffering, and death, which no amount of artificial physics will eradicate. We must learn the lesson now. Already it may be too late, and every day sees man's natural environment violated by the pollution of our soil, water, air, and even the very kernel of our being.

CHAPTER VIII

Effects of Drugs on Eyes

"I have cured granulations of the eyes, in chronic conjunctives, by Hygienic treatment, after all kinds of drug applications had failed".

Prof. W. Parker, M.D.

That drugs in any form are dangerous and can cause more damage than is usually admitted has been the standpoint of all health reform movements. It is therefore encouraging to find a book written by two pharmaceutical chemists—*Drugs With Possible Occular Side Effects* by H. Green and J. Spencer—who admit that some common drugs in day-to-day use for the so-called common day-to-day illnesses can cause appreciable damage to one of the most delicate organs in the human body, namely the eye. Dr. L. J. Fish, who recently read a paper at a medical congress in Brighton, which was subsequently printed in *Clinical Trials Journal,* draws a picture so horrifying that any complacency on the part of the medical profession to continue to use drugs instead of natural care of their patients is nothing short of criminal.

Judge for yourself, if in order to alleviate your aches and pains you are willing to pay a much dearer price—that of losing your vision or impairing your vision in any way.

The so-called anti-cholingeric drugs, including belladonna and atropine, have beeen known to cause dry mouth and blurred vision in 48% of the patients who took these drugs for the treatment of peptic ulcer. The purpose of using this class of drugs in the treatment of peptic ulcer is to reduce gastric secretions and motility, which are initiated by impulses from the vagus nerve. This nerve is part of the parasympathetic nervous system which, of course, has many ramifications throughout the whole body and carries out its work in exactly the same way in all of these regions. Hence, it is not only secretomotor to the stomach, but it has the same function to the salivary glands. After swallowing the drug, it is absorbed into the bloodstream and then carried around the body, where it has an anticholinergic effect, which means it blocks nerves that secrete acetylcholine. Similarly, it achieves its effects in the eye by blocking the parasympathetic impulses there, and the patient has a dilated pupil and loss of accomodation, and complains of blurred vision. It follows, therefore, that any patient taking any kind of anti-cholinergic drug may be expected to complain of blurred vision when he is on such drugs. Let us consider together a few drugs in common use and their known effects in impairing or destroying vision.

Corticosteroids: These drugs are very widely used and have dramatic effects in certain diseases. The drugs are used both systemically and locally in the eye and, of course, topically on the skin.

The effect on eyes and vision of steroid therapy, both topical and systemic, involve "allergic reactions"; viral, fungal or bacterial infections; ptosis; dilation of the pupil; modification of refraction; papilledema; optic neuritis; cataract; ocular hypertension leading to glaucoma; and about ten others difficult to classify, including retinal hemorrhage, thin transparent or blue sclerotics and granuloma. Conclusion: Patients on prolonged topical or systemic steroid therapy must have regular eye examinations, in which attention is particularly directed to the lens, the disc, and ocular tension.

Quinine, chloroquine and hydroxchloroquine: Quinine is well known to produce regularly toxic visual changes which are bilateral, sudden in onset, and capable of progressing to such an extent that there is a marked constriction of the retinal arteries and some degree of atrophy.

The anti-malarial drugs which were derived from quinine were developed during the Second World War. They are now used in the treatment of rhumatoid arthritis and have been known to cause keratitis and retinopathy.

Corneal deposits: Toxicity due to synthetic antimalarials was first reported from the U.S.A. in 1946, following observations on airmen taking mepacrine. One year later a British factory doctor reported a similar toxicity in workers engaged in manufacturing the drug. When Hobbs and Calnan reported their findings in the Lancet in 1958, the patients' visual complaints included blurred or misty vision, difficulty in focusing, sore eyes, and colored haloes around lights. The haloes were particularly noticed when driving at night. Twenty-two out of thirty patients examined had corneal changes. The trouble was confined to the epithelium of the cornea, with some slight changes in the stroma immediately under Bowman's capsule in a few patients. Some had irregular, white, linear deposits with dotted additions; in some there was a yellowish color to the deposits, in others the dots were gathered into curved lines, giving an appearance like a magnetic field of force. Corneal deposits disappeared when the drugs were stopped.

Retinopathy: This group of drugs has been known to cause severe retinal pigmentary degeneration, with loss of vision, peripheral contraction of the visual fields, attenuation of blood vessels, pigmentary changes at the macula, and sometimes peripheral changes. The changes are *not* reversible and in fact, may progress after the drugs have been withdrawn. In 1966 Arden and Kolle reported on a country-wide survey of 347 patients suffering from rheumatoid arthritis, who were receiving anti-malarial therapy. The overall incidence of retinopathy was 13%. The results of their observations are particularly important in that they indicate the early signs of toxicity.

During prolonged chloroquine treatment, they state, abnormalities may appear in the fundus while the patient's vision is still unaffected. The earliest change is slight pigmentary mottling of the macula and in the perimacular region. Later, retinal and subretinal edema occurs with definite pigmentary changes producing a "bull's eye" appearance. In one case this was followed by loss of visual field as a true retinopathy developed, suggesting a stage of pre-retinopathy which might be recognizable. If this is so, and if drugging is stopped, progress of the disease might be arrested before irreversible changes occur. The toxic effects of these drugs rose to 40% in those whose total dose exceeded 86/Kg body weight. The steroids and the anti-malarials have been dealt with in some detail because they appear to be of great interest and importance as so many people undergo this type of drugging. Other commonly used drugs that induce occular toxicity will now be mentioned briefly.

The contraceptive pills have been the subject of anxious

comment in both the lay and medical press, since they became available. In America the Federal Drug Administration (F.D.A.) saw fit to issue a statement warning of possible eye toxicity. The resulting troubles may include: double vision, retrobulbar neuritis, and thrombosis of the central retinal artery. The F.D.A. also insists that the labels on the packs of these tablets should carry a warning referring to the "optical hazard".

Sulphonomides and phenylbutazone, especially the long-acting ones, may precipitate the Stevens-Johnson syndrome—a condition involving the skin and mucous membranes throughout the body. The ocular (eye) complications include pseudomembraneous conjunctivitis, leading to symblepharon and scarring of the lids (which may be severe), and corneal ulceration followed by scarring and loss of vision.

Phenylbutazone may also produce retinal hemorrhages and the sulphonomides may induce myopia. Certain sulphonomides have been reported to produce unwanted effects on the lens, which may be an allergic edema. Sulphonomides have also been known to cause conjunctival and scleral congestion, giving the appearance of pink eye, with burning, smarting, and watery discharge. The condition is aggravated by exposure to light. The Phenothiazine-chlorpromazine drugs have been reported by several authors to cause oculocutaneous changes seen in those on long-term high-dose treatment. All were women with mental illness, and the doses were from five hundred to fifteen hundred milligrams daily for three to ten years. In one series, twenty-one out of seventy patients were severely affected. The toxic changes described were: purplish pigmentation of the eyelids; diffuse corneal haziness, and small central lens opacities.

The corneal lesions are described as wihte or yellowish-white fine specks in the stroma, these being especially in the deep and central areas. (This is in contrast to chloroquine which affects the epithelium of the cornea). The lens opacities are stellate, central and in the anterior subcapsular region (again, one may note in contrast that the steroid-induced cataract occurs in the posterior subcapsular area). Chlorpromazine has also been reported to cause papilledema; toxic amblyopia, retinitis, and pigmentary retinopathy.

Other tranquilizers: Thioidazine, a phenothiazine derivative, has been shown to produce pigmentary degeneration in the retina. Some of the tranquilizers have atropine-like side-effects and should not be given in the presence of increased ocular tension.

Monamine Oxidase Inhibitors: Pheniprazine ('Cavodil'; Carbon' in the U.S.A.) was reported in 1958 to be the cause of red/green color vision deficiency, which was reversible on stopping the drug. A subsequent report in 1960 stated that when some of the patients were 'challenged' with resumption of treatment, the color defect recurred, together with altered visual fields. Optic atrophy had also been reported in connection with the use of this drug. The drug was subsequently withdrawn from the market.

Carbromal: This hypnotic is available (amongst 16 other preparations containing it) as a capsule which contains carbronal and pentbarbitone. A man of 42, who had been taking these capsules at night for five years, found he had blurred and double vision. Stopping the capsules himself, he found an improvement after three nights. When he restarted treatment, the visual symptoms returned. He reported to his doctor, who found he had bilateral lens opacities; the corrected vision was 6/6 and 6/9. The treatment was stopped, and two weeks later the vision was 6/5 with each eye. Ten days later there were no lens opacities on examination.

Anti-epilectics-Troxidone: Troxidone has also been reported for some time to be a cause of photophobia and the 'glare phenomenon' with blurring vision when the eyes are exposed to a bright light. This occurs mainly in adults and develops during the second week of therapy. The condition is reversible on discontinuing the treatment. Phenytoin sodium, which is one of the drugs very commonly used in epilepsy, may also cause blurred vision, diplopia, and ptosis.

Antibiotics: Chloramphenicol—a wide-spectrum antibiotic—has several times been reported as producing optic neuritis. In 1956, a Japanese author described two cases of retrobulbar neuritis in patients who were having systemic treatment. The eye toxicity was preceded by generalized peripheral neuritis, including weakness of accomodation. The adverse effects occurred some fifteen to twenty weeks after beginning the treatment. Both patients showed a deficiency in vitamin B6 uptake, suggesting that this might be secondary to the antibiotic therapy.

Isoniazid, with streptomycin and PAS, used in pulmonary tuberculosis, has been reported to be the cause of optic atrophy, sometimes followed by blindness. The incidence is rare, and the neurotoxicity has been connected with the giving of high doses into the cerebro-spinal fluid surrounding the spinal cord, in the treatment of tubercular meningitis. Unfortunately, the illness itself is a cause of optic atrophy and blindness, but more than one author has reported that the incidence increases with the giving of isoniazid by the intrathecal route. Isoniazid may also produce an allergic reaction of the face and eyelids, involving the conjunctiva, with visual disturbances such as blurred vision. Optic neuritis, followed by optic atrophy and ocular palsies, has also been reported.

Ethioamide has rarely caused optic neuritis and photophobia. Ethambutol has been reported to cause a decrease in central visual acuity and severe amblyopia in some patients. Impaired color vision has also been noted. Amphotericin B, one of the newer antifungal antibiotics, may cause deterioration of vision. Streptomycin may produce scotomata and blurred vision, due to C.N.S. effects. Kanamycin may also cause blurring of vision and optic neuritis, and coliston has caused transient visual disturbances.

Antidiabetics: Both Insulin and chlorpropamide may produce hypermatropia via an electrolytic change which affects the lens. The latter drug has also been reported to cause bilateral central scotomata with marked visual loss. This is reversible on discontinuing the treatment.

Ganglion blocking agents: These are widely prescribed in the treatment of hypertension. They can cause either a paralysis of accommodation, or a spasm of it resulting in myopia.

Digitalis: This is also a commonly prescribed drug being used in cardiac diseases, and it may produce visual disturbances by action on the higher centers. The changes include foggy vision, altered color vision, wherein objects appear green, yellow, or white (as if covered with snow), diplopia, and sometimes blindness. These visual symptoms may be present whilst other (peripheral) toxic effects are not. The disturbance in vision is reversible on withdrawal of the drug.

Diuretics: The benzthiazides are now well-known to cause diabetes mellitus. They may also be the cause of transient myopia, particularly in pregnant women. Acetazolamide, used in glaucoma, may provoke a reversible myopia.

Anticoagulants: It is easily understood that these drugs may cause subconjunctival hemorrhage, which is described as usually harmless. Patients receiving them carry a card describing their treatment.

Oddments: Two reports may cause one to be on the lookout for the unusual. Firstly, the local use of two percent pilocarpine in a 75 year old man, according to an American report, produced a systemic toxicity. Secondly, another American author related the loss of pigment from the skin, in the region of the eyelids, in four negroes, with the use of eserine (and other drugs) in the treatment of glaucoma.

Experimental Toxicology: The alleged value of the present system of animal studies, followed by human clinical trials in which particular attention is paid to possible toxicity, is claimed to be borne out by the story of dimethyl sulphoxide (DMSO). The chemical is a well-known indusrial solvent, produced as a by-product in the manufacture of cellulose. In 1964 two American research workers published their findings, indicating a wide range of potential therapeutical uses for DMSO. These included—penetrant carrier; local analgesic; anti-inflammatory agent; bacteriostat; diluretic and tranquilizer.

Unfortunately, the lay press gave wide publicity to the drug in colorful terms and, even more unfortunately, the crude industrial solvent (rather than the refined substance used in research) began to be used by private persons who were suffering from rheumatism and muscle strains, etc. Many of the original claims for DMSO failed in critical clinical tests, but the drug continued to look extremely interesting as a carrier (through the skin) of other drugs. However, in November 1965, and almost simultaneously from one British and two American research units, came reports of animal toxicity in three species, in which a change in the refractive index of the lens was noted. The lens change followed both oral and topical dosage, and was time-dose related. Such changes had not been observed in humans, but the six American drug firms involved, after discussion with the F.D.A., sent telegrams to their clinical investigators to stop clinical trials and withdraw the drug, pending further investigations.

Cataract after tranquilizers: Two Hungarian opthalmologists, M. Varga and P. Jabbagy, have recently reported cases of cataract associated with the use of tranquilizer therapy. The specific drug was Quietidin, a piperazine derivative. The reports concerned ten patients who developed photodermatitis and then cataract in the posterior lens cortex. Stopping the medication checked progression of both conditions. Other Hungarian doctors have found similar consequences. One of these suggests that decomposition of the drug may upset the chemical balance of the organism, as a result of which there may be a breakdown in resistance to detrimental or excessive exposure to light.

Intensive research is recommended on the incidence of cataract development following excessive administration of tranquilizing drugs. We suggest discontinuing the use of the drug.

Another drug with terrible effects on the eyes was reported in the Chicago Daily Tribune, January 1963, with headlines, "Miracle Drug Found Cause of Blindness". The report says that "the synthetic drug chloroquine, which has worked medical miracles in certain illnesses, has been implicated in 26 cases of creeping blindness". The report also informs us that "the drug is the synthetic quinine which was used by the ton to check and prevent malaria in American armies in the tropical battlefields of World War II . . ." The drug slowly destroys the retina of the eye—probably like arsenic, producing optic atrophy. The field of vision in cases investigated was narrowed and narrowing in a similar pattern while spots of destroyed vision were present in varying sizes.

Another equally disturbing report is to be found in the Manchester Guardian, May 11, 1967: "Drug Could Damage Eyesight" ran the headline. "Delegates at the Northern Optical Congress in Harrogate were told of the sideeffects of a drug used to treat arthritis and malaria. It could have disastrous results and do irreparable damage to the eyesight, said a member of the Pharmaceutical Optics

Committee, at present studying the harmful optical side effects of drugs".

Bibliography: "The Ophthalmic Optician" 20th July and 10th August 1968; "Drugs Affecting Vision" by R. Hertzberg in the Medical Journal of Australia, 1965.

CHAPTER IX

Drugs and the Nervous System

"The science of medicine is a barbarous jargon and the effects of our medicines on the human system, in the highest degree uncertain, except indeed that they have destroyed more lives than war, pestilence, and famine combined".

John Mason Good, M.D.F.R.S.
Author of "Study of Medicine"

The nervous system of man is a highly complex thing in itself. It is more so than any other animal, and because it is a highly complex mechanism, for the same reason it is also very sensitive and delicate in its structure and function.

This highly specialized system acts very quickly and shows sometimes immediate and marked changes if in any way changes inimical to its well-being are made. Drugs can and do influence the structure and function of the whole nervous system.

Driving, for example, requires skill and steady nerves, especially in our day and age when almost everyone uses a car even to go a block round the corner. "Don't Drug and Drive" is a warning given by "Drive", the motorist magazine of January 1969 issue. According to this article, alcohol and drugs are not conducive to the safe usage of so powerful an instrument as the modern motor car. The reason given is that the person's reactions are influenced by the bodily changes that are undergone when alcohol and drugs are imbibed.

The writers infer from their investigations that some two million motorists in Britain drive regularly under the influence of drugs, and they quote, in support of their contention, the fact that in 1967 family physicians wrote out more than 271 million National Health Service prescriptions for drugs, which included 20,900,000 for sleeping tablets, 14,700,000 for tranquilizers, 4,900,000 for anti-depressants, 4,800,000 for stimulants and appetite suppressants and 5,100,000 for antihistamines. They point out—as we have been doing all along in this book—"that a large number of drugs in daily use produce side-effects . . . varying from mild dizziness to outright collapse . . . which may seriously undermine driving ability. Even cough syrups, stomach powders, and aspirin can produce dangerous effects. Yet the harsh fact is that, up to now, nobody in Britain has attempted to relate the effects of drugs—physical impairment, personality change, and the like to motoring".

The article is well authenticated and also gives a table of the known side-effects which those drugs, freely prescribed by physicians, are likely to have upon their takers. As an example of the possible side-effects which anti-depressant drugs may cause, we quote from the chart in "Drive": "Palpitations, blurred vision, defective color vision, agitation, diminished self-control, anxiety. Particularly dangerous in combination with alcohol, many other drugs, and some foods like cheese, yeast extracts, broad bean pods, etc. Effects with any of these range from headaches to collapse and sudden death".

Thoreau, the American Philosopher, once said that for the thousand who were hacking away at the branches, there was only one striking at the roots. This certainly applies to much of today's medical practice, where a great deal of attention is given to the effects of disease, but very little to its causes.

If the nervous system goes haywire, it needs freedom from noise, hustle and bustle of the rat race, stimulants and sedatives, alcohol, coffee, tea, chocolate, "cokes" and such-like social poisons, and not "remedies" out of the chemist shop. The right kind of mental attitude, a positive approach to life, physiological, mental and emotional rest, sleep (not coma of narcotics) and such-like are nature's needs for recovery of health.

That the nervous system gets a tremendous amount of beating when drugs are taken is now consistently shown in reports such as follows. Under the headline, "Side-effect of Medicine", the London Times, October 19, 1966, wrote: "The physical and mental handicaps which were taking the place of infectious diseases were speech defects, blindness or partial sight, deafness or partial deafness, epilepsy, physical handicaps, maladjustment and educational sub-normality. Asthma appeared to be increasing".

Thus, in trying to cure the so-called infectious diseases of the children, the medical profession is destroying the health and well-being of the nation's childhood. Prof. Rene Dubois, the Rockfeller scientist, once said, "One of the most neglected aspects of the germ theory of disease is the fact that infection rarely produces fatal disease under natural circumstances".—a point worth remembering before rushing out to your physician if little Johnny has a cold and fever.

Another report from the London Evening Standard, April 12, 1969, goes to show that drugs taken for so-called nervous ailments are in themselves producing and perpetuating the very same conditions they are trying to cure. "Drug Warning by Doctor" is the headline and report: "Self-poisoning by people swallowing over-doses of barbiturates, tranquilizers, anti-depressants, and hypnotic drugs has now reached epidemic proportions in Britain, a leading expert said today. And the total of these cry-from-the-heart patients is rising. Dr. Henry Matthews of Edinburgh's Royal Infirmary, told the British Medical Association's annual clinical meeting that, unless the epidemic was stopped, the whole of the population of Edinburgh would need treatment for drug poisoning by 1984 . . ."

✦ This is certainly a frightening position but we must again remind ourselves that all these drugs are on prescription, and that the obsessional attitude of taking drugs for the cure of ills is largely to blame for the present orgy of medicine taking.

A change has to come, and the sooner the medical profession realises it, the better it is. To supplement the above comment, we quote a report from the London Times, April 12, 1969: "Dr. Cubson warned against a prevailing belief that careless prescription was the prerogative of some other doctor. They should look repeatedly at the haphazard way in which they tended to use penicillin and antibiotics; at how they could create chronic malingering by weekly certificates for symptoms which the patient started to use as an excuse for staying at home; *at how they uncritically prescribe sedatives and hypnotics for a high percentage of patients month after month, to create a degree of drug dependence which would shock even a most hardened statistician if the figures ever came to light; and how they played their part in producing drug poisoning and death".* (Italics K.R.S.) This places the responsibility just where it belongs.

*Many people are under the false impression that vaccines and immunization shots are not drugs but, if we look at our definition of the word Drug in the very beginning of this book, we will see that drugs can be of animal origin. For all practical purposes, vaccines, serums, etc., are all poisons and classed as drugs.

The Manchester Guardian on March 19, 1969, reported that a well-known drug company had suspended its supply of the measles vaccine and had given the following reasons for so doing: "This decision was taken because of recent reports of a few isolated cases of complications involving the central nervous system, which arose in children within about eight days of vaccination . . ." The report continued: "The company said there had been three cases—including one death—where the children aged between one and two had contracted encephalitis after being vaccinated. The disease occurred in about one case in 3,000 of natural measles, and also after a smallpox vaccination".

May we add that many such reports can be quoted where polio vaccine has been given and the victim paralysed as a result of such tampering with nature rather than from poliomyelitis.

The present craze of heart transplants, apart from being futile where heart disease is concerned, brings added difficulties to the unfortunate victim of such tom-foolery. Both the London Evening Standard, May 7, 1969, and the Daily Telegraph, May 8, 1969, had disturbing headlines about the effect of heart transplantation. That in the former said, "Heart-swap patients who lost their minds", while, according to the latter, "U.S. heartgraft patients become mentally ill". The report went on to say that, according to Dr. Donald T. Lunde, psychiatric consultant to the heart transplant team at Stanford University Medical Centre, California, 5 out of 13 people who had received hearts at Stanford became psychotic after the operation. In the same report, we are told that "the use of the drug Prednisone, one of the drugs used to counter the rejection mechanism of the body, is also known to affect some people mentally". . . . Here we must emphasize that the whole transplant technique is a great shock to the system, but we believe that "nervous symptoms" which are prevalent are due to the anasthetic drugs, as well as other drugs which are pumped into the body before such a transplant can take place. The overall guilt is once again of the drug poisons violating the sanctity of the human body.

This is an age of neurotics, and so-called "nervous diseases" and nervous instability are symptoms of a lack of emotional poise. The old Hygienists used to have a slogan, "Be Poised or Be Poisoned". It is good to see, therefore, that an eminent authority like Dr. Edmund Jacobson, Director, Laboratory for Clinical Physiology, Chicago, and the Jacobson Clinic, writing on the subject of "Anxiety and Tension Control" seems to agree with this slogan. He says: "Evidence is presented illustrating that the more we teach our anxious patients sound knowledge, personal self-control and the know-how to live in emotional security, notwithstanding the many difficulties to which they need to adjust, the less we need to rely on medication. The results can prove rewarding both to the doctor and patient, compensating them for the time necessarily devoted to educaional procedures. In contrast with the problems *that attend the use of drugs, there is reason to believe patients who are taught to do without drugs will be better off in the long run.* Since emotional reactions are of primary significance, not only in function but also in many organic conditions, it seems reasonable to expect that much of scientific medical practice of the future may well be in teaching the patient to do for himself".

And we say 'Amen' to all that. So many people suffering from "nervous disorders" ruin their lives by drugs. We have known of cases where epilepsy has been perpetuated by drugs to control the convulsions. Sleeping tablets and tranquilizers are habit-forming and do nothing to induce sleep, which is a normal function of life. Instead, they dope the body into a state of semi-consciousness or unconsciousness and actually prevent sleep—so that a greater dosage becomes necessary as time goes by to bring them to the stage of coma-like unconsciousness. People habituated to taking sleeping pills and tranquilizers always feel "hazy in their vision and fuzzy in their head". Their reactions are slow and inco-ordination exists in their movements. Sometimes even voluntary control of speech is affected.

John C. Button, Jr., M.D., in his book, "Hope and Help in Parkinson's Disease", observes that Parkinson's Disease is common among individuals who are treated with tranquilizers for other conditions. It is definitely stated by Button that in a small minority of patients, permanent Parkinsonian states may be induced by drugs. He further states that it is not rare at all for one to develop Parkinsonism while on tranquilizers for mental disorders, saying that as many as 38.9 percent of patients out of 3,775 have presented symptoms of Parkinson's disease, while being dosed with tranquilizers. This is especially true of the tranquilizers of the phenothicizine group. Other known chemicals and drugs that cause symptoms of Parkinson's disease (a disorder of the central nervous system) are the barbiturates, carbon monoxide, carbon disulphide, and manganese.

And yet drugs are given to "control" Parkinson's disease. The victim is abused to death by drugs. To squash symptoms, such a large dose is necessary in some cases that side reactions become a problem. Then a drug is given to squash the side reaction of the first one. For example, an antihistamine such as Benedryl causes drowsiness and to compensate for this, a stimulant is given, such as Amphetamine.

Artane, a medically popular drug used for Parkinson's Disease, supposedly loosens the muscles and calms the tremor and excitement. Its toxic reactions are confusion, restlessness, hallucinations, dryness of the mouth and throat, and blurring of vision. Other side reactions from the many drugs used in this disorder are mental confusion; slowing of bladder function; skin rashes; aggravation of existing glucoma; dizziness; indigestion; nausea; vomiting; restlessness, and delirium.

The contraceptive pills so freely prescribed have been known to cause severe headaches, epileptic seizures, and cerebral acclusive incidents (hemorrhages) according to David B. Clark, M.D., Professor of Neurology at the University of Kentucky, as reported in the Philadelphia Inquirer for April 29, 1966.

It is practically impossible to exaggerate the evils of the drugging practice, but every time we think we have added up their evils the drugging profession hauls out yet another list of damages they are producing with their poisons, and we have to start all over again. Anybody who understands the relations between drugs and the living organism knows that it would break a law of nature (and her laws are inviolable) for a drug to give rise to anything other than an evil effect. It is impossible for them to do good. Forrest Adams, M.D., Professor of Pediatrics at the University of California, admitted way back in 1965 at a lecture when speaking at a luncheon at Statler Hilton Hotel, in aid of the United Cerebral Palsy Association of Los Angeles, California, that chances of babies suffering brain damage at birth are increased by the widespread use of pain-killing drugs by mothers during pregnancy and childbirth. Adams reported that three out of four babies born prematurely suffer with cerebral palsy. If this is so, is it not a recent development? Was it true 50 or 100 years ago? Is it true in Sweden and other parts of the world where mothers are not drugged?

A letter in Medical News, August 27, 1965, tells of effects of nalidixic acid, saying that: "the exact incidence of reactions is difficult to assess, but between May 1964 and April 1965 there were reported to the Committee 52 cases of skin rashes and 126 cases affecting the nervous systems in patients being treated with nalidixic acid. Between January 1964 and February 1965 general practitioners alone issued approximately 77,000 prescriptions for the drug". The reactions were described as follows: "visual disturbances, excitement, depression, confusion, and hallucinations have been reported. Headache, giddiness, drowsiness, syncope and sensory disturbances have also occurred in a few instances. One patient had a grand mal attack which might have been due to the drug".

Once again, we should try to remember what a teaching member of an American medical school wrote in the Lancet, August 19, 1961: "It would be naive to believe that the pharmaceutical industry exists in order to advance science, cure disease, or promote humanitarian good will; these are only incidental by-products of their very clear and natural aim to make profits and sell their wares".

Let us now see some of the common drugs used for so-called "nervous disorders" and what effects they have on the nervous system.

Bromide is a typical drug and used very frequently. Apart from the notorious "Bromide Acne", the effects on the central nervous system are psychic disturbance, headache, mental dullness, lethargy, difficulty in concentration, abnormal behavior, confusion, hallucinations, delirium, and even full-blown psychosis. The commonest neurological symptoms are slurred speech, ataxia and tremor (of the hands alone or generalized). (from "Side Effects of Drugs", Vol. V., by L. Meyler 1963-65).

Barbiturates are freely prescribed in our pro-drug society. The same author as above states: "Drowsiness, dizziness, and headache are not uncommon after-effects following the use of a barbiturate as a hypnotic. Particularly in the elderly, confusional states have been attributed to the barbiturates". In the same book, we find on page 36, "Drugs with a depressant action on the central nervous system are used in large quantities at the present day, and increasing numbers of nonbarbiturate sedative drugs are being introduced into medical practice. These preparations are, however, not only extensively used but also widely abused. Addiction, psychical or physical dependence, chronic and acute intoxication, the latter either accidental or resulting from attempted suicide, are well-known problems. Despite claims to the contrary, nearly all the drugs belonging to this group can cause addiction . . . Linked with the depressant effect upon the central nervous system is the influence upon pulmonary ventilation. Ventilation and respiration can be markedly depressed by these drugs, and in patients with previously impaired ventilation this side-effect may be disastrous."

It must be very difficult for those who know nothing about Natural Hygiene or "Nature-cure" to understand how one can live without medicine, and equally difficult for nature cure advocates to understand how anyone can expect to be fit and healthy when he is taking into his system substances that are highly toxic. The barbiturate drugs are a good case in point. They are hypnotic sedatives which have no curative value even in the conventional sense of the term, and their safety is very variable depending on dosage. The book, "Drug Induced Diseases", now in its fourth volume in 1975, lists nearly twenty adverse effects which the barbiturates may have on the body and mind, and it reveals: "It was estimated that the total number of cases of barbiturate poisoning in 1959 was nearly 10,000, and that the quantity of barbiturates prescribed by general practitioners in the National Health Service had doubled between 1953 and 1959 from 81 to 163 thousand pounds".

The consumption of these drugs still goes on apace. The Minister of Health, as reported by the Times (October 31, 1975), appealed to doctors to make sensible savings in prescribing such drugs: "In 1972 in England more than 45 million prescriptions were written for such drugs at a cost of nearly £23 million, and similar figures were recorded for 1973 and 1974. The overall trend for such drugs continued upwards". Now, after all these years, there is a movement among some medical authorities to place certain restrictions on the use of these drugs so as to prevent such colossal over-use.

Apart from sedatives and tranquillizers, other drugs known as stimulants or anti-depressant drugs are the most commonly prescribed drugs for "nervous disorders". "Caffeine" habitually taken in chain-drinking of one cup after another of coffee is a well-known culprit, causing nausea, nervousness, insomnia, and sometimes increased diuresis, even in average doses. In large dosage, to the above symptoms one can add vomiting, tachycardia, extra systoles of the heart, insomnia, restlessness, nervousness, tinnitus, tremors, and scintillating scotomas; also prolonged hydrochloric acid secretion leading to perforation of duodenal ulcer in a man.

The other well-known stimulants and anti-depressants are the amphetamine derivatives (purple hearts, green hearts, goof balls) and the M.A.O.I. (Monoamine oxidase inhibitors), the former causing euphoria, psychic disturbances, restlessness, inco-ordination of thought, insomnia, irritability, hallucinations, anxiety states and suicides; the latter causing serious liver damage and marked hypotension (hydrazine group) and dangerous hypertensive crises with increase of blood presure and sometimes even intracranial bleeding (tranylcypromine group). The nervous system is also affected when taking cortico steroid drugs so commonly given in arthritis and other rheumatoid conditions.

In general, administration of corticosteroids may cause mild euphoria. Sometimes, however, more marked psychic changes occur, and agitation, confusion, mania, hallucinations, and full-blown psychosis have been described. Psychotic conditions may be accompanied by fear or depression; suicides in this condition have been reported. Such psychic symptoms may occur after oral, parenteral and even topical application of corticosteroids. An increase in the number of epileptic seizures or the relevation of a latent epilepsy have been described during use of corticosteroids". (L. Meyler, Side Effects of Drugs, page 407).

Prednisone and triamcinolone are the most popular in this range.

The antibiotics are as guilty as any other drugs for upsetting the nervous system. "Penicillin has an irritant action when applied directly to the central nervous system. Elecroencephalographic abnormalities and convulsions occurred after application of penicillin solution to the human cerebral cortex. Signs of penicillin irritation (increased neuromuscular irritability with muscle twitching, hyper reflexia and convulsive seizures) may occasionally appear in patients with uremia when the combination of high parenteral dosage and impaired excretion result in a very high plasma penicillin concentration". (L. Meyler, page 293).

"The most important and serious side-effect associated with the use of streptomycin, and more especially of dihydrostreptomycin, is the toxic damage to the 8th nerve, which may occur.

Vestibular disturbances and deafness are not uncommon. Dizziness and tinnitus sometimes precede vestibular dysfunction or deafness, but often no such warning symptoms occur".

Certain other neurological effects have also been reported. Dizziness, tinnitus, paraesthesia, flushing and paralysis of the eye muscles may occur. Ocular muscle paralysis may sometimes be seen in combination with nystagmus". "Streptomycin has been found to have a blocking action on neuromuscular transmission, causing severe muscle weakness". (L. Meyler, Side Effects of Drugs, pages 297 and 298).

Once again we must bear in mind the Thalidomide tragedy, when talking about drugs and the nervous system. D. G. Friend, M.D., in an article, "Drugs and Fetus" in January 1963 issue of Clinical Pharmacology Therapeutics, says that, "Although considerable information has accumulated concerning the passage of drugs through the placenta and their effect on the fetus, unfortunately little attention has been paid to this aspect of drug therapy, and on the whole, there has not been any concerted effort to bring this type of information to the attention of physicians. However, the recent Thalidomide episode has stirred up a great deal of interest in this phase of pharmacology".

Drugs with a molecular weight of 1000 or less are known to usually succeed in passing the placental barrier. Drugs like Tubocurarine, a muscle relaxant, anti-spasmodic and convulsant, easily passes to reach the fetus and more significantly, it has been found that many agents which ordinarily do not pass through the placenta will do so if the patient is toxic.

These phenomena are similar to that which happens in a severe central nervous system infection. There are clear cells in the central nervous system called protoplasmic astrocytes, whose function is to guard brain cells by keeping out certain inimical substances. This is called the blood brain barrier. However, in the presence of a severe central nervous system infection, this barrier breaks down and allows penicillin, which normally does not readily pass the barrier, to reach the nerve cells.

Morphine and Meperidine (Demerol) are the most extensively used narcotic analgesics. Indeed babies have been born, as said before, addicted to morphine as a result of the mother's addiction. Many babies are born with a typical pin point pupil caused by morphine addiction in the mother. Others are dangerously cyanotic (blue) from anoxia, due to severe depression of the respiratory center in the brain, from the use of morphine only in delivery.

Phenacetin, another analgesic extensively used, and contained in many patent medicines like Bromo Seltzer, besides causing addiciton to the drug, produces disturbances in the central nervous system, liver damage, methenoglobincina, sulfhemoglobinemia and anemia. While taking large amounts of phenacetin-containing drug, a young pregnant woman developed metheglobinemia and sulfhemoglobinemia (a state in which the hemoglobin cannot be oxygenated and therefore is equivalent to an anemia of comparable degree). If she was taken off the drug after developing these states, evidently damage to her unborn child had already been done, for it died of degenerative encephalopathy one month after birth.

Tribromoethanol, once widely used for obstetrical anesthesia, besides depressing the mother's nervous system, also deeply depresses the nervous system of the fetus. After its use as a basal anesthetic during labor, newborn babies were found to remain inactive for almost a week after delivery.

Having seen so many thousands of people who have been sick for years, and who failed to get well with regular and the most skilled drugging by qualified orthodox medical physicians, most of whom have made immediate gains in health when drugs were discontinued, we are naturally skeptical of all forms of drugging. There is far more drug addiction in the world than is commonly recognised.

Way back in 1916 (long before the author was born) the first edition of "A Layman's Handbook of Medicine" by Richard C. Cabot, M.D., of Harvard University, was published. In this book Cabot says: "Eighty percent of the people who have the morphine habit in this country have acquired it from doctors. So Dr. Alexander Lambert states in "Osler's Modern Medicine". Eighty percent acquired it because of drugs given them by physicians. I think on the whole, the greatest single evil I know I know in medicine is the abuse of opium and morphine. . . . I stated that eighty percent of the cases known to Dr. Lambert were due to the opium given in prescriptions by physicians.

A considerable portion of the remaining twenty percent are doctors themselves. The profession which figures most numerously in the list of occupations of those who get morphinism is the medical profession . . ." If however you, dear reader, think that the picture has changed in this jet and space age, you have a shock coming.

A few years ago, in 1965, the London Sunday Telegraph, under the heading, "Shock Report on Drugs", said: "Mr. Robinson, the Minister of Health, is about to receive a shock report on the gravity of drug addiction in Britain. The report from Lord Brain, the neurologist, and a committee of seven eminent doctors, will be the first ever made to government naming addiction to hard drugs as a major problem in Britain". Apportioning the blame for the great prevalence of drug addictions, the Telegraph says: "It lays the blame for the growth of addiction to morphine, heroin, and other drugs squarely on the medical profession. The report says over-prescription by doctors is the only source of supply".

Also under the title, "Troubled Doctors Hooked on Drugs", is a report by Sid Katz in the Toronto Daily Star, May 29, 1965, which asks, "Why do so many doctors become drug addicts?" Katz says that the "best available estimates suggest that drug addiction is 30 to 100 times more prevalent among doctors than among the general populaion". He adds that "if the addiction rate among the general population were the same as that of the medical profession, then we would have in Canada about 200,000 drug addicts to worry about, instead of about 3,500".

And in the magazine "Parade", of April 25, 1965, a ten-year study of 107 doctors' wives admitted to a phychiatric home showed that forty-one of the total number were started on drugs by their husbands. It is a sad commentary that 37 of the women were registered nurses.

A few years ago, in 1965/1966, we read about the death of a young man who had become addicted to sniffing glue. He had first sniffed the glue for "kicks". Then the habit grew until he could not stop it. His mind became cloudy, thinking was difficult, he couldn't remember things, and he was dull and sluggish. He was made mentally ill by the fumes of the glue. This did not happen overnight but slowly over a period. His brain was damaged. This is a conspicuous example of cause and effect. But when Hygienists say that you can go crazy by chronic poisoning, we are not listened to.

But the medical profession has begun to realize, as in Boyd's Textbook of Pathology 1961, that what we stigmatize as mental illness and insanity is simply a biochemical disturbance of nerve cells, manifested by impaired synaptic transmission of an impulse. Mental illness can thus be attributed to the very drugs given by the medical profession.

Bromide is one example. Since the discovery of methods to determine the amount of bromides in the blood, some twenty years ago, physicians have discovered that more people than they realized were being placed in mental institutions with insanity due to bromide intoxication. As high as 4 percent of all people in some mental institutions were there with a psychosis, which developed because of taking drugs containing bromides. And it is stated that physicians were directly responsible for fifty percent of these cases by prescribing the drug. Noyes and Kolb, in their book, Modern Clinical Psychiatry, state that "All too frequently, additional amounts of the drug are further given in an effort to rid the patient of symptoms already caused by bromides".

Cortizone and ACTH both directly affect the brain and produce mental disturbances of many opposite and varied types, from joviality and optimism to depression and hypomenia, and apathy to panic. Delusions, illusions, and hallucinations may be experienced. Recovery takes place when the patient is taken off the drugs before the damage to the brain has been done.

In the past few years Isoniazid has been used in treating tuberculosis, and physicians have noted a number of psychotic states developing from its use. In these cases the patients are completely disoriented for time, place, person, and situation. They have auditory and visual hallucinations. The drug also causes constipation and difficult micturation.

Chronic barbiturate intoxication produces symptoms similar to a very serious disorder of the nervous system, namely Multiple Sclerosis. There will be involuntary rapid movements of the eyes (nystagmus), impaired speech, muscular incoordination, and a loss of the superficial reflexes. In severe intoxication, the patient falls into a coma from which he cannot be aroused; there is a complete absence of all reflexes and manifests the symptoms of shock.

Other drugs causing mental symptoms similar to those produced by cocaine, are the sympathomimetic amines, such as Benzedrine, Dexedrine, and Desoxyn. Sulfanamides (sulpha drugs) also produce mental symptoms. Thiocynates produce mental symptoms, as well as mercury, manganese, lead, carbon monoxide, carbon disulfide, belladonna, chloral hydrate, and paraldehyde. Delirium has developed occasionally even from the introduction of atropine into the eyes. We must remember that no drug can be taken without causing some trouble somewhere in the body, and the central nervous system is affected by most of them.

Tybamate, a tranquilizer, has some 20 different side-effects attributed to its use in the 1966 edition of New Drugs, with the following under the heading of precautions: "Patients receiving Tybamate should be advised not to undertake activities that require mental alertness, judgment, and physical co-ordination."

We must bear in mind the words of Lt. Col. Robert H. Moser, a physician in the Army Medical Corps, uttered in a symposium on "Diseases of medical progress", as reported by True Magazine of June 3, 1966, which prefaced a devastating indictment of the drugging business by an incongruous descriptive heading "Helpful but Harmful". This is what it said: "The wonder drugs of modern medicine have carried a high price tag and the bill keeps getting bigger . . . *patients are paying it with an increased number of drug-induced diseases*". (Italics mine, K.R.S.)

Moser made a most telling statement of fact when he admitted, "Although each drug is designed to act upon a particular organ or upon particular tissues, we are inclined to forget that the drug is also in contact with other tissues—effects in those areas are not immediately evident—subtle influences may be at work and may become manifest only later . . . "Such long range effects, he warned, "may never be traced to the drug that caused them". He also admitted that penicillin causes many deaths a year and also that the effects of certain drugs are not limited to one generation.

That a great majority of people who choose to commit suicide finally do so by taking barbiturates and other depressant drugs is not commonly known. The Drug Trade News of November 8, 1965, carried an account of a symposium on suicide at the George Washington School of Medicine in Washington, D.C., in which the use of drugs to end one's life was discussed.

It was disclosed that rauwolfia and its extracts—serpentina, resperpine, and other alkaloid derivates of this tranquilizer "are particularly suspect" as leading some patients to attempt suicide. This is because reserpine occasions emotional disturbances manifested by the patient's withdrawal from his environment, together with feelings of lethargy and unhappiness. It was indicated that this mental depression is more likely to develop if the drug is administered in large doses for a month or longer. After discussing the varying views of medical men, Frank M. Berger, M.D., said, "I feel that the bulk of available evidence indicates that rauwolfia alkaloids are more likely than any other central nervous system depressant drug to produce depression and lead to suicide".

In spite of all this knowledge, the medical profession goes on blundering with drugs with the excuse that the good done outweighs the harm done by drugs. We regret that we do not see any good done by the taking of drugs. As we have said repeatedly, drugs only mask symptoms but do not remove the ultimate cause of disease, namely toxaemia.

However, it is good to see that here and there the hygienic stand on the uses of drugs may not be altogether unwelcome.

For example, in a book "Drugs in our Society", (edited by Paul Talalay, Johns Hopkins Press, Baltimore, Maryland, published in 1964), we read the following by Maxwell M. Wintrobe, Professor of Medicine and Chairman of the Department of Internal Medicine, University of Utah College of Medicine. He comments: "The desire to take medicine is the greatest feature which distinguishes man from his fellow creatures. This observation, attributed to William Osler, is as true today as it was in the dark ages of history. Unicorn's horns, crocodile dung, Egyptian mummy and sarsaparilla, not to speak of simple remedies such as animal or human urine, have all had their days of popularity. The more horrible, the fouler smelling, the more revolting the remedy, the more impressive and, in some situations, the more effective it was.

"In our modern society, medicines are dressed in more appealing forms, and they are often introduced with such promise and fanfare that the expectant public daily anticipates the working of miracles. Furthermore, there are remedies for every complaint and they are consumed in large quantities. *Some members of our modern society behave as if life were a process of existence which can barely be maintained or endured without taking a continuous series of wonder drugs*". (Italics mine, K.R.S.)

But who is responsible for conditioning the public in this matter, if not the physicians and pharmaceutical industries, we ask?

Who has made the public so dependent on drugs that they now tell the physicians what prescription they want, we ask? The professor cannot pass the buck to the people— the responsibility for such a state of affairs in our mind lies solely with the medical profession and the drug industry.

He continues: "The adverse reactions problem is not new; only the attention given to adverse reactions is recent. The problem attracted the attention of the informed medical world in the early twenties, when Werner Schultz in Germany identified a dramatic disorder which was given the name "agranulocytosis". He described a syndrome characterised by the sudden onset of sore throat, prostration and fever, often followed by sudden death, in formerly healthy people. Those affected were often women of the well-to-do classes. Examination of their blood revealed a marked leukopenia with a total absence of granulocytes. In time, it was shown that this syndrome was associated with the taking of a newly introduced analgesic, amidopyrine".

"The problem did not die with the incrimination of amidopyrine. A familiar pattern has been repeated over and over again. A new drug is introduced. It is vaunted highly. It is used widely and its sales increase rapidly. Ill effects are encountered here and there. They multiply. Ultimately, the news is disseminated, the use of the drug lessens and, in the end, the popular drug may become a "drug on the market". As other remedies appear, the pattern is again repeated".

This is what the Hygienist has said for 150 years or more, but now it appears to be authenticated. However, the most striking statements to which we want to draw the attention of you, the reader, is what follows. The Professor continues: "There is a mistaken impression on the part of some who lately have become aroused about the problem of drug reactions that the testing of drugs in a sufficient number and variety of animals will provide the information which will call attention to adverse effects of drugs, and will thereby protect prospective human recipients. While it may be true that in certain instances more adequate laboratory tests should have been carried out, and in others clues concerning possible adverse effects were ignored for various reasons, nevertheless it must be recognised that laboratory tests cannot eliminate completely the risk involved in the taking of drugs. Accidents due to toxic reactions in man *will continue to occur as long as drugs are used. There is an element of risk with every drug that is prescribed".* (Italics mine, K.R.S.)

These were the unanimous conclusions of a panel of

experts who met together at the second International Pharmacology Congress in Prague in the summer of 1963".

Reader, you have been warned. You will not know what is happening to you until it has happened, when you start taking drugs—prescribed or self-prescribed.

CHAPTER X

Drugs—Your Liver and Alimentary Canal

"Every dose of medicine administered to a sick person should be seen as an admission of defeat on the part of the practitioner. For a doctor to drive back a symptom without uncovering its cause is malpractice in one of its more hazardous forms".

J. Seate (Any Change is Progress)

Some 30 years ago it used to be said that if a patient visited ten physicians, he would obtain ten different diagnoses and ten different kinds of medicine, the excuse being that medicine was more of an art than a science. Today we are assured that modern medical knowledge has raised it to a science, but we have our doubts. The reason is not far to see. The London Daily Mail, September 30, 1967, with a feature article, raises considerable doubt in our minds as to how much progress has really been made.

The article deals with the treatment of peptic ulcer and was based on the report of the Sainsbury Committee, which has been looking into the question of Health Service drugs. It showed that a sample of 463 doctors were asked the question: "What would you prescribe for a patient suffering from peptic ulcer?", and it turned out that no less than 45 medicines might be used to treat the same complaint. "They include capsules, tablets, liquids, and gels. They vary in price from less than a half-penny to more than seven pence an ounce for liquids and from one shilling to 18 shillings (in old money) a hundred for tablets".

In this age of mass-medication and controversies of public health, can the layman resist pressures brought on him in the name of "science" while critical scientists may be muzzled or misquoted? To make matters worse, physicists and chemists are often ignorant of biology, and do not suspect or want to suspect what effects their discoveries could have on man and his surroundings.

All the blessings of science we enjoy are the fruit of individual schemes of trial and error, intellectual tussle and adventure. Not only war can endanger further progress, but also peace and prosperity, if they bring sloth and refusal of responsibility. It is the ignorant and irresponsible whose craving for a magic solution puts tyrants into power. Racial magic did not free the German people from their hysterical fear of encirclement; it made their condition worse. Magic stones and pills will not help the masses who have been talked into a morbid preoccupation with their diseases and ill-health, but may damage their health by delivering them into the hands of medical demagogues. Safety from ill-health is the subject of this book. The following words and pages are written to think of safety in a versatile manner.

So-called safety measures are imposed or accepted on the promise or in the hope that they will prevent the occurrence of some form of bodily harm; safety thus rests in the future, it exists in the form of predictions. One has to act now if the promise or hope is to be fulfilled later. All promises and hopes are not equally justified, and we clearly need a guide to estimate the value of predictions. This is particularly important in this century when promises of good health are widely used for the promotion of political and business interests, e.g. fluoridation, the most recent brain-child of the medical and dental profession.

The safety of man owes much to instinct. Through millions of years of evolution, the line of existence that eventually emerged as man was preserved by instinct and through the good fortune of circumstances not beyond powers of endurance. With the appearance of rational man, our dependence on instinct and environment lessened. Intellectual power exercised some control over both our environment and instincts.

Not so many years ago the individual had a chance to look after his own safety, irrespective of the community's views on the subject. Today, at least in the most advanced countries, it is difficult to think of individuals in a state of biological independence of the group. Air, water and food are all affected by military, industrial, and agricultural techniques. Radio-active fallout from northern experiments affect the southern hemisphere. Insecticides and weed killers are carried by the wind and in the products treated by them.

Immunization, regular exposure to radiation or national service demanding the handling of highly dangerous materials, are often enforced by law.

In many countries of the world the worship of "health" is served by an increasingly powerful branch of the Civil Service and by the privileged members of the medical and dental professions. In an anti-clerical age we, the public, are becoming subject to the new monks, priests, and prelates of a disease-serviced profession; our respect for their saints also adds power to their inquisitors.

One could argue that the "fight against disease" justifies the emergency powers conceded to the witch doctors—old and new—but there are some valid objections to this view.

Few individuals are accustomed to rational thought, and a little pressure is enough to make most of them accept group ethics. The thinking minority may be repelled by group ethics, but the divided loyalty which results has dangers of its own. One of these is the tendency of loyalists or conformists to obstruct individual thinking and criticism by fair means or foul. This happens in Fascist, Nazi, or Communist-governed countries. It is less commonly appreciated in countries with ballot boxes that mass education by propaganda through the press, advertisement, and broadcasting monopolies is directed against the rational and responsible individual. Although safety as canvassed in arguments by orthodox medicine is usually treated in terms which seem to be concerned with the natural sciences, often in fact are a travesty of them, e.g. fluoridation. One of the tasks of the Hygienist is to detect the anti-rational background of some of these arguments.

Laymen have as much right as scientists to worry about their safety. They have not only the right but the ability to sort out the true, imaginary and fake varieties of evidence used to woo their votes.

The material rewards of science are so plentiful that new discoveries are taken for granted, and the part played by searching is no longer appreciated. Thus, science—which is a mode of searching—is rapidly becoming a magic word to settle an argument. Science as the name in which we are urged to accept other people's views, medicine, waste products, and meddlesome care is a false god which must be destroyed if reason is to prevail.

Another item in the British Medical Journal of January 27, 1968, entitled "Drugs and the Liver", is a case in point, that no part of the human system escapes damage and deterioration from the taking of so-called safe drugs.

The liver is a great detoxifying organ in the human system. There is a saying, "Is life worth living?" and the answer, "It depends on the liver" is not as far-fetched as it seems.

Medicines are, of course, foreign agents so far as the body is concerned, and when they are taken into the system, their toxicity has to be neutralized or reduced by the function of the liver. The liver stands as a sentinel, and if for any reason the liver should fail in its important function, the economy of the body is greatly disturbed. With the discovery and development of the more powerful drugs, the liver is placed under a very great strain.

The article says: "The last quarter of a century has seen the introduction into clinical practice of large numbers of new and potent therapeutic agents. Many of them have unexpected effects on the liver, which sometimes have little clinical significance but which may be fatal. Many of the hepatic sequelae, and unfortunately most of the serious ones, cannot be predicted on the basis of previous tests of toxicity on animals. The rarity of some and their close resemblance to naturally recurring acute viral hepatitis may make it difficult to identify the drug with the untoward reaction".

Drugs and alcohol are perhaps the worst offenders in putting strain on the liver, with insecticides, pesticides, chemical preservatives and so on, on our food nowadays, as a close second.

In relation to the damaging effect alcohol has on the body a recent report in the British paper "Sunday People" of March 14, 1976, states: "Don't Drink to Love". "A report from New York: Don't ask a man to drink and make love. They just don't go together, according to doctors here who have been researching the problems of sex and the drinking man. They report that alcohol forces the liver to produce excessive enzymes which can eliminate the male sex hormone testosterone. Dr. Emmanuel Robin says: our research over many years, show men have a choice—drink or women".

Kasper Blond, an eminent enlightened physician, quoted in a book "A Cancer Therapy" by Dr. Max Gerson, says: "The whole syndrome of metabolic disorders which we call oesophagitis (inflammation of the oesophagus), gastritis, duodenitis (inflammation of the duodenum), gastric and duodenal ulcers, cholecystitis (gall bladder inflammation), pancreatitis (inflammation of the pancreas), proctitis (rectum inflammation) and others, are considered only stages of a dynamic process, beginning with liver failure and portal-hypertension (hardening of the blood vessels which provide the liver with its circulation) and resulting in cirrhosis (hardening) of the liver tissue, and sometimes in cancer".

᠂ Dr. Boyd in his book "Pathology of Internal Disease", stresses the same point. He says, "the cells of the liver are bathed in the blood brought by the portal vein from the gastro-intestinal tract, blood which may contain toxins known or unknown. The result of such toxic action may be the death of some or many of the cells of a liver lobule; it may be of one or many of the lobules themselves" . . . . . Dr. Boyd is quite specific in saying what these toxic materials are which have a destructive effect upon the cells of the liver. He says: "Among the numerous agents, most diverse in character, which may cause degeneration and necrosis of the liver cells may be mentioned chemicals, *both organic and inorganic, certain drugs and tarlike substances, foreign proteins and products of protein decomposition, bacterial toxins, injections and exposure to radiation"*. (Italics mine, K.R.S.)

Let us take note of the fact that Aspirin, Anacin, Pyramidon, Phenacetin and the Sulfa drugs so freely prescribed by physicians are coal-tar derivatives. No doubt the liver gets worn out and damaged. Dr. Fenton Schaffner of the Department of Medicine and Pathology, Mount Sinai Hospital, in a report presented before the section on Gastroenterology and Proctology at the 109th annual meeting of the American Medical Association, pointed out that "Jaundice induced by drugs may be the result of hepatocellular damage (damage to the liver cells), cholestasis (stoppage of bile flow), or hemolysis (breakdown of the blood)".

This report, taken from the Journal of the American

Medical Association, November 26, 1960 (Iatrogenic Jaundice) quoted Dr. Schaffner as also saying, "As therapeutics progressed from galenicals to complex chemicals which profoundly affect many biochemical reactions in the body, iatrogenic diseases have become more numerous. The liver, because of its central role in metabolism and excretion of many drugs, is a frequent target of an untoward and unexpected action of a drug".

An important point that was stressed by Dr. Schaffner and which we would like to emphasize, is that the liver symptoms occurring from the use of a drug show after some delay or may not turn up until after the patient has been taking it for weeks, or even up to a month after its administration has been discontinued.

Let us say here quite emphatically that the medical profession and especially their High Priests of the calibre of Sir William Osler, Professor René Dubois, and Louis Pasteur and Dr. J. Wendel MacLeod, all are aware that a healthy body builds its own immunity to so-called "infections". The irony is that in actual practice this point is in most instances tragically overlooked or disregarded. Osler, in his "Practice of Medicine", says, "the human individual in normal health is practically immune to natural infection, and only when the body is in a depleted condition, can an infection develop". Should we then not pay attention and learn how not to deplete our life's energies, we ask?

Louis Pasteur, in the later stage of his life, was also evidently aware of this, since, according to René Dubois (in "Mirage of Health"), he pointed out in his writings, "that the response of the infected individual was determined by his hereditary endowment, his state of nutrition, his environment including the climate and even his mental state" and, whilst studying the disease of the silkworms" came to the conclusion, startling for the time, that the micro-organisms present in such large numbers in the intestinal tracts of the silkworms were *more an effect than a cause of disease*".

We also heartily endorse the words of Dr. J. Windel MacLeod, Dean of Medicine, University of Saskatchewan, as reported in the New York Times, September 2, 1959: "Large sections of our people clamour excessively for x-ray examinations, chemical tests and surgical procedures", concluding, "confidence in the healing power of nature has been displaced by undue dependence upon the popular drugs of the moment".

But once again, we ask who helped the lay public to lose confidence in Nature, if not the physicians and their drugs? Why is there nothing being done by the medical profession to restore this confidence? Who protects the drug industry, and why this double dealing?

That a drug like Aspirin used for over a century and whose misdemeanors include causing gastro-intestinal bleeding, impaired blood-clotting, anaemia, and fatal allergic response as the acetic acid is transferred to body proteins, and more recently that the drug can destroy enzyme activity, is still prescribed by physicians, is proof enough of our statement that the medical profession may be indulging in subterfuge and double dealing.

The stomach is the first line of defense when taking drugs orally, and has been known to be damaged in one way or another. For example, Dr. M. S. Israel told Medical News (November 4, 1966) after the Erasmus Wilson Demonstration at the Royal College of Surgeons of England, "Salicylates (aspirin), phenylbutazone and oral cortisone drugs can cause local erosions of the gastric mucosa by direct contact with the tablet".

Indigestion is one of the most common symptoms that has plagued mankind, and especially so in our modern civilization.

Whether the symptom be heartburn, sour stomach, bad taste, halitosis, loss of appetite, belching, nausea, vomiting, cramps and discomfort, or feeling of fullness in the abdomen, constipation—all are danger signals warning us that attention is necessary and that we should do something to remove the cause of the trouble. The trouble may be the use of irritating substances in our diet, e.g. spices, condiments, rich food, extremely hot or cold foods, and social poisons like, tea, coffee, alcohol, chemicals, and drugs.

Or it may be a symptom of general toxemia, where the metabolite toxins generated by the body in normal wear and tear do not have the opportunity to be eliminated and voided by the body, or it may be nervous or emotional tension causing temporary malfunction of digestive system, or it may be our wrong habit of eating "foodless foods"— demineralized, devitalised, doctored, and dead foods, or it may be our faulty eating habits—not enough mastication, voracious eating, gluttony, eating when not hungry, eating when ill or emotionally upset, wrong combinations of foodstuff, and many more reasons that one could think of.

But instead of analysing the trouble and admitting our faults, we rush to the physician or the nearest drug store to get an Alkaseltzer or sennapods, or castor oil, or acid-neutralizing tablets, or any of the other myriad compounds devised by those who firmly believe that a symptom suppressed is synonymous with recovery of health.

The result—not only perpetuation of the disease with its periodic symptoms, but chronic degenerative diseases, due solely to the habit of taking such poisons in the guise that they are medicines because they are prescribed by a physician.

We cannot give a better proof than the statement made by Dr. Gordon McHardy of the Brown-McHardy Clinic and the Department of Medicine, Louisiana State University School of Medicine, in a paper read before the General Scientific Meeting at the 107th Annual Convention of the American Medical Association on June 24, 1958. He said: "The most widely used and probably most effective therapeutic agents today have been responsible for dramatic gastrointestinal reactions that have introduced new entities (of ailments) into the medical literature. Thiazine-induced cholostatic jaundice, anti-biotic resistant staphylococcic, pseudo membraneous enterocolitis, and steroid-activated or steroid-produced peptic ulcers have each offered frustrations to the therapist whose agent boomeranged so as to product another illness".

He went on to say: "The gastrointestinal tract is exceptionaly susceptible to untoward reaction to certain therapeutic agents" and, naming digitalis, colchicine, atropine as well as those given specificaly for digestive disorders like chlorpromazine, iproniazid (marsilid), the arsenicals, the rauwolfia compounds (tranquilizers), A.C.T.H., cortisone, and other cortisone-hormones, the anticholinergies (those that inhibit the flow of secretions and the action of the digestive organs) as well as the opiates.

Taking of bicarbonate of soda to relieve acidity of the stomach has become both a myth and a legend in our lifetime. However, "all that glitters is not gold" and, similarly, it is so with such measures. In his book "Treatment in General Practice", Harry Beckman in evaluating this procedure cites one study which showed that in one half of the patients examined, this remedy "caused a rebound in gastric acidity to a point higher than would have been attained had the alkali not been administered".

Discussing this point further, he quoted Steigman and Fantus to the effect that the reduction of acidity through the use of such methods is neither great nor long-lasting, and may be followed by a rebound increase.

In the Sunday Observer of January 1, 1956, we find under the heading "Antibiotics warning to Doctors", an article which corroborates the basic argument of Natural Hygiene. "Chlortetracycline and oxytetracycline are so effective against bacteria that they kill off helpful germs which are normally present in the digestive tract. As a result, disease-causing fungi may grow unhampered and the building up of essential vitamins by the intestine's bacteria may be interfered with. Worse still, killing off harmless germs may allow other pathogenic germs, which are normally suppressed, to flourish, sometimes with fatal results".

At the British Medical Association Annual Meeting of 1967 it was pointed out that 30 percent of all illness was due to the unnecessary and wrong use of drugs, and that 20 times more antibiotics were prescribed than was necessary. One thousand deaths a year were attributable to the wrong use of antibiotics.

Diarrhoea is not in itself a disease but an action of the body against some form of toxic irritation mainly from unsuitable or unhygientic foodstuffs. Holidaymakers travelling abroad are most likely to suffer in this way and it has long been the custom to use drugs as counteracting agents. The Guardian (July 8, 1975) carried the headline "Diarrhoea Drugs May Be Lethal", and the British newspaper covered a recent report on them: "The report says that anti-diarrhoea drugs can cause kidney and liver diseases, skin and sight defects and even death . . . that clioquinol-based drugs have reached the stage of folk remedies, that none of the trials over the last forty years have shown clioquinal is effective against diarrhoea . . . diarrhoea should clear up on its own and should not require the taking of drugs . . .".

Thus, Nature is never fooled—the more you suppress

the symptoms, the greater the struggle by nature to warn of impending danger and, if still not heeded, it continues struggling until, weary of struggle, depleted of its vital energies, it gives up the struggle and succumbs. Death then is not due to disease but to the unequal struggle that the body has to wager continually against crimes committed in the name of wonder-cures and wonder-drugs.

In the words of Dr. Shelton, "Perhaps no other thing has cost mankind more pain, misery and real suffering than the idea that he should poison himself because he is sick".

CHAPTER XI

Drugs and the Circulatory System

You and Your Heart

"You and your heart—no-one else,
Knows the secret of your dreams,
The heights of your ambitions,
The depth of your degradation.

You and your heart—no-one else,
Probe the weakness of your strength,
The strength of your weakness,
And balance the two.

You and your heart—no-one else,
Can sacrifice the temple of your body
To gluttony, gold and greed
For disease, disenchantment and death.

You and your heart—no-one else
Must decide now
A way of life or else
Stand by for time to stop,
Because you and your heart are one."

(From Words & Music and All Alone
by K. R. Sidhwa.)

It was Herbert Spencer who declared that mankind never tries the right remedy until it has exhausted every possible wrong one.

We are forcibly reminded of this statement when we read how well known and so-called harmless remedies are beginning to lose their prestige value because of the harm that has been found in their wake.

We all know that during the war and even before, cod liver oil for infants and Vitamin D were No. 1 on the list as welfare foods for the young. In 1957, however, cod liver oil became suspect, so much as that The Lancet of April 29, 1961, carried some remarks by a doctor at the Royal Hospital for Sick Children. After discussing the casual role that it might play in infants' troubles, he carried on: "Nevertheless, Vitamin D and cod liver oil have also been found to cause poisoning in children and may, moreover, cause heart lesions. Myocardial lesions and electrocardiographic signs suggestive of them have been attributed to cod liver oil medication in early childhood . . ."

The Hygienists have said all along of, all those articles which are not utilized and appropriated by the body to be a part of its constituents, that such an article is not a food but a poison. Where is the logic of those who now wish to prescribe cod liver oil as an anti-cholesterol agent?

The very drug that is supposed to be of benefit has been found eventually to be the culprit that does harm in the long run. For example, for many years the drug Digitalis, derived from the common purple foxglove, has been in widespread use as a heart stimulant, so-called. Formerly it was used by monks and laymen for other troubles, including tuberculosis, until taken over by medical men, who did so when W. Withering discovered its use as a heart stimulant. From the very first days, it was realized that it produced very different reactions in individual patients, and great trouble was taken to arrive at a uniform dose. In Britain "the unit of potency is defined as the quantity required to stop the heart beat in an anaesthetized cat; in the U.S.A. the unit is defined as the quantity required to kill a frog of 25 grams weight".

However, its dangerous nature (as of all other poisons) was given an airing in a report in the British Medical Journal, May 8, 1965: "A recent paper by Schoff is a timely reminder of this and is full of good sense about the use of this potent drug. In an analysis of 2,000 consecutive electrocardiograms recorded in a hospital group, he found that 12 percent of those patients, who had recently had Digitalis, had records suggesting excessive dosage. Thirteen patients died within a period of the last electrocardiograms, and in nine deaths it was considered to have been directly due to, or at least accelerated by, Digitalis".

Another clipping from an American newspaper stated: "Digitalis drug poisons many patients". The article states: "Digitalis, one of the most commonly used drugs for treating heart failure, causes some form of poisoning in an unbelievably unusually high proportion of patients who take it". This article was published in 1969 and quotes John Ruedy of the McGill University, who blamed it on improper use. May we ask, improper use by whom, if not the physicians? Could there ever be a proper use of a substance that is a poison? Drugs damage and lessen the vitality of every organ and organ system in the body.

When a drug is given to a man suffering with a weak heart, it weakens the heart still more. It is like whipping a tired horse to make it go. The impaired heart must now pump more blood with each beat to help get the drug out of the system by increasing circulation. But the heart, in doing this, will wear out more quickly than if left intelligently alone and the patient allowed to rest. The heart needs rest, not stimulation. Exhaustion of all the vital organs is the common result of such stimulation.

Flogging the heart with digitalis, strophantus, quinadine, caffeine, or other poisons is a stupid and harmful practice. Sedation of an excited and rapid heart is as stupid as stimulation for a weak or slow heart. Sedatives are depressants. A heart sedative not only abates the force of the heart's action, but the vigour, and the rate of the heart's action is reduced. Among the cardiac sedatives are listed such poisons as aconite, antimony, chlotal, chloroform, conium, the nitrites, tobacco, and others. All of these produce damage to the heart.

In an article, "Digitalin Intoxication", Dr. Arthur M. Master quoted Von Jaksch, who in his book on poisons stated, "Digitalin and digitoxin are frightful cardiac poisons. Their use at the bedside necessitates the greatest care. A single excessive dose of these glycosides invariably results in death from cardiac paralysis in a short time". (Journal of American Medical Association, June 5, 1948).

Paul Dudley White in his book, "Heart Disease", although extolling the virtues of digitalis, points out: "Auricular paralysis, auricular fibrillation, various high grades of heart block, a coupled rhythm due to ventricular premature beats every second beat, idoventricular rhythm, ventricular paroxysmal tachycardia and ventricular fibrillation have all been induced in man or in animals by massive doses of digitalis . . . when any of these disorders of cardiac mechanism are found to result from the digitalis given and not primarily from other factors, the drug should be discontinued, for a high percentage (50 to 90 percent) of the lethal dose has probably been given by the time such disorders are found".

Levine, in his book, "Clinical Heart Disease", also states "Therapeutic doses of digitalis produce no pathological changes in the heart muscle; toxic doses do cause definite necrosis of the heart muscle fibres and inflammatory changes and also changes in brain cells". By therapeutic dose, Levine means "35 to 40 percent of the lethal dose". However, the basic fact that all drugs can be accumulative is disregarded by physicians, and damaging effects only come to light eventually. However, a significant comment by Dr. White, in his book, proves that the precaution they (the physicians) take is delusory. He states: "The toxic and therapeutic effects of various preparations of digitalis or of other drugs of the digitalis series are parallel; *a preparation that can be taken in large dosage without toxic effects is apt likewise to be therapeutically inactive and a preparation that is very active therapeutically tends quickly to cause toxic symptoms*".

Thus, you cannot have it both ways—a poison can never be safe and not be a poison. The danger is inherent in its being.

Mercurial diuretics so frequently prescribed in congestive heart-failure also have a history of morbid fatality.

In the New York State Journal of Medicine, October 15, 1949, there is an article by Dr. Leon Merkin, stating the dangers from the use of this drug, "Among the side-reactions, the most important is the death of the patient shortly after the injection". Killing them to cure them is one way of removing disease, it seems.

Tetany, uraemia and, in some cases, stupor, are some of the other side-effects that occur from the use of these drugs.

An editorial in the Journal of the American Medical Association, November 17, 1951, seemed to confirm this viewpoint, stating, "Although congestive failure itself predisposes to thrombosis (a closing of a blood vessel) there is some evidence that this tendency is aggravated by currently accepted therapy for congestive failure, and particularly by the injudicious use of mercurial diuretics".

The nitrites (nitroglycerin and amylnitrite) are used for angina pectoris to give dramatic relief. But they force the heart to work harder and help to dilate the arteries—the relief obtained at the cost of greater enervation and fatigue to the heart. Doctors know that the body's oxygen will combine with the nitrites, and its availability for functional use is reduced. Thus a vicious circle is established. Besides, none of the drugs help to strengthen the heart and improve its vitality and function.

The present fanfare of "wonderful drugs" used as anti-coagulants is also on the wane. As long ago as April 22, 1961, in an editorial entitled "Possible Risks in Anti-coagulation Treatment of Cerebral Vascular Disease", the Journal of The American Medical Association reported the findings of neurologists in nine Veterans Administration Hospitals covering the observations of 155 patients, in half of whom anti-coagulant drugs were used for an average period of about nine months. It states: "Not only was the incidence of recurrent cerebral infarction apparently un-altered by anticoagulation, but treated patients had a higher mortality than controls (those who did not receive anti-coagulant drugs). The increase in deaths was due partly to the occurrence of cerebral hemorrhage, a complication which has been observed in other studies, and which is regarded as a major risk of this therapy".

One realises that thickened blood must be thinned, but it is one thing when this is accomplished by following a diet regimen, or fasting, that helps to bring about this change, and quite another when it is done with a remedy that tampers with the coagulability of the blood.

Some years ago the "New York Medicine" of May 1949 stated a case of Dr. Ernest Klein, who was discharged from his position at the Bellevue Medical Centre, New York University because he published the result of his findings that a diet of fresh orange juice diluted in water and noth-ing else will help to thin thickened blood. And yet Levine in his book states that a semi-starvation diet diminishes the work of the heart and produces other favorable effects on the circulatory dynamics. Which would you choose— to fast and rest and eat moderately and wisely to recoup your health, or go on asking for relief all the rest of your life?

In 1962, at their medical conference in Belfast, the members of the medical profession heard Professor John McMichael of London University denounce the use of anti-coagulant drugs. To quote the Daily Telegraph, he said: "bluntly, that treatment with anti-coagulant drugs, the aim of which is to reduce blood-clotting, should cease. The risks of treatment were considerable, and the risk of death was always there. One is producing a bleeding disease in order to stop clotting. Patients have had to be withdrawn from trials because anti-coagulant drugs caused severe brain damage".

"With this treatment there was a possible death rate of up to four out of ten patients for a possible gain of six lives. The ones who died were not necessarily the ones who would have died, untreated, from thrombosis". In the discussion that followed, Professor McMichael demonstrated, as the others had done before him, a lack of follow-through that we find curious, if not heart-breaking. For example, when one of the doctors present said, "I am 33 and moderately fit. I know how to avoid getting my ulcer. What measures must I take to avoid getting my coronary?", the Professor's reply was, "I hope the doctor chose his parents well and that they are long-lived. The only other thing I can suggest is that he should pray and put a little reliance on statistical evidence".

This then is the difference of approach between Natural Hygiene and the medicine man of today or of yesteryear. In other words, no emphasis on preventative measures. As the witch doctors of old cast a spell upon us, so our complex civilization of today will hurl a thrombosis at us. Such would seem to be the Professor's philosophy. No suggestion of more exercise or less food, or of avoiding emotional strain or any other things that can harm. Such then are the high priests of the medical profession, whose statements, like the books they write, bear little resemblance to the practice which is carried out from day to day.

At the same session of the British Medical Association, a leading physician asked the heart specialists who were on the speakers platform what they would do if one of them were to be suddenly "struck down" by a serious myocardial infarction. The replies are revealing. Professor Theodore

Crawford (pathologist) replied: "I would like to have no treatment at all".

Tage Hilden, M.D., a Danish expert, replied: "I would not take anti-coagulants". Sir George Pickering, Professor of Medicine at Oxford University, said: "When I have mine, I hope treatment will not be necessary. I am 58, and I think that the evidence that anti-coagulants do any good for people over 55 is so small that I would not want any".

Professor McMichael said that if it was a small infarct, he would stay in bed for a few days and not tell anyone; if it was a medium-sized infarct, he would go to bed and call his general practitioner; if he were collapsed and shocked, he would agree to being admitted to a hospital, but he would like to choose the physician looking after him. He would, however, much prefer not to have anti-coagulant treatment.

Hilden and McMichael both discussed statistics of cases treated with and without anti-coagulants and came to the conclusion that so far as recovery and survival are concerned, there is no significant difference in the two modes of treatment, which to us would indicate that their non-coagulant therapy is also bad. But Hilden stated that bleeding occurs more often in anti-coagulant treated cases, and necropsy hemorrhage into the pericardium (the investing membrane of the heart) was more common in those receiving anti-coagulant treatment. He also stated that he had discontinued using the anti-coagulants.

McMichael stated that there is really no indication that can be taken as incontrovertible for the continuance of the use of the anti-coagulants. Such therapy, he stated, is dangerous, ineffective, and a burden to the physician, the patient, and the laboratory, and it should be discontinued. More than 12 years have now passed since the famous meeting and, while these eminent physicians and heart specialists agreed that the anti-coagulants are dangerous and ineffective, the anti-coagulants are still being freely manufactured and prescribed all over the world.

Why continue the dangerous practice?

Nearly 22 years ago the British Royal Society of Medicine announced, "anti-coagulant treatment of coronary occlusion will go the way of other discarded remedies it is certain; let it go soon, let it go now, before remorse weighs too heavily on those who may continue for a little time longer to advocate its use".

What is wrong with a profession that can continue a mode of treatment after it has become convinced that it is ineffective and dangerous, even at times lethal, we ask?

Reading the magazine "Look", (December 31, 1963), we find in it an article by Dr. Morton F. Hunt on "Iatrogenic Diseases" in which he notes, "Heart disease of electrocardiographic origin is perhaps the commonest and most serious".

In Hygienic circles we consider mass radiography to be a mistaken procedure, doing a great deal of harm for a small and problematical advantage. Hunt underlines the situation in these words: "Many new, improved diagnostic procedures introduce a small degree of risk. A patient enters a hospital . . . and runs a gauntlet of such tests, and the little risks add up".

Hunt notes, "The basic principle in medicine for many centuries was *'Premium non nocere'*—'First of all, do no harm'—but we have almost forgotten it today", and he was quoting the words of a doctor after a young woman patient had died within minutes of taking an antibiotic injection for a sore throat. It is surely no pious complacency to point out that the principle of doing no harm is very much alive in Hygienic practice.

Another way of expressing it is that we do nothing to a sick person that we would not do to a healthy one. Indeed, we carry the idea much further and consider it essential to treat the ailing individual with a gentleness to match his lack of vigour. As Dr. Herbert Shelton so truly emphasises: "The weaker the patient, the greater the need to do nothing". In case the reader should think that we are making too much of this point, let him reflect that in orthodox medicine it is routine to use the most powerful—that is the most poisonous—drugs in the most seriously ill cases.

Let no-one imagine that the modern wonder drugs are any less toxic than the old-fashioned varieties. Hunt goes on to say: "Thalidomide is not alone; many other useful drugs being administered by doctors today may damage unborn children. Vitamin K can cause blood disorders. Sex hormones may prevent miscarriage, but can cause half-masculinised sex-organs in baby girls. Certain sulfa drugs can cause degenerative nerve disease. Anti-psoriasis drugs can cause gross physical deformities in the unborn child".

Hunt also notes the following miscellaneous effects:
"Hundreds of cases of aplastic anemia—nearly always fatal
—caused by chloronycetin, others by some of the tranquilizers commonly used in mental hospitals. Nausea, headache, weakness, skin irritations, baldness, and anemia can
all result from excessive dosing with vitamins, especially A
and D. Blindness—retrolental fibroplasia—results from
prolonged administration of pure oxygen to a newborn
baby".

We hear so much at the present time about open heart
surgery and the undoubted high technical skill which ac-
companies it, that there seems to be little room for discussion about the factors which may make it necessary.

To suggest that drug therapy may in some cases be
responsible in this way may, to some people, seem to be
straining the imagination, but the following, taken from
Health For All, December 1968, needs no obvious comment: "Dr. Leonard Lorshin, of the Cleveland Clinic, has
supplied information concerning a 30 year old woman in
whom, after six months of methysergide therapy for headache, marked aortic regurgitation and a myocardial infarct
developed. Open heart surgery performed by Dr. Efflet
revealed a thick fibrotic ring involving the root of the
aorta and the orifice of the left coronary artery. The aortic
valve leaflets were thickened and incompetent and were
replaced by a prosthesis".

Also, "Clincal observations show that the heart is more
frequently involved as a shock organ in cases of drug
allergy than had previously been realised. Changes in electrocardiograms resembling cardiac infarctions, angina pectoris and myocarditis may develop . . ."

A recent report in the paper "The Guardian" (April 24,
1975) says: "Doctors were warned yesterday to avoid
using a leading heart drug because of the serious side
effects it can cause. The warning came from the manufacturers of the drug, 'Eraldin', which has been used by more
than 250,000 people since it was introduced in 1970". This
shows that in spite of the most conscientious testing of
medicine by manufacturers, the last experiment must be
made on the patient.

That drugs damage the blood and the blood-making
mechanism is confirmed in an article by John Troan,

Scrips-Howard Science writer from Washington, March 21, 1962. He tells of a "study-group" of the American Medical Association and how they have linked 48 drugs and a variety of blood diseases. The drug-induced diseases ranged all the way from a mild anaemia to a "vicious type of aplastic anaemia which is usually incurable".

Chloromycetin—an antibiotic—was indicated as the number one culprit and "seemed to have a definite toxic action on the bone marrow, where blood cells are made".

The American Medical Association Committee listed the following of the better-known drugs which have shown or are associated with blood dyscrasias:—Antibiotics—Chloromycetin, Ristocetin, Streptomycin and two of the anti-B drugs, including PAS (Ristocetin is said to be employed against staphylococus germs); Tranquillizers—Meprobamate (Miltown and Equiani), Thorazine Pacatal and Aprine; Sleeping Pills—Sedromiel (a pep-up pill to fight severe mental depression) and Tofranil.

Anti-arthritis and Antigout drugs—Colchicine, Butaolidin, Benemid and gold salts; Pain-killers—four, including Phenacetin; Anti-Diabetes pills—Orinase and Albinese; Anti-stimulants—Diamox, Diruril, and Furadantin; the first two are employed in reduce blood pressure, the third is employed in kidney "infections".

Anti-coagulants—Phenidone and Quinidine; the first is described as a heart smoother; the second is said to regulate the heart beat.

Anti-epileptic drugs—Dilantin, Methoin, Mysoline, and Tridione.

Thyroid drugs—The Thiouracils, Thiobarbital, and Methimazole.

Sulfa drugs—Six, including Kynex, Protalbin, and Gantrisin.

Well, dear reader, which one is your favourite poison? More extensive testing of drugs before putting them on the market and greater caution in administering them are not the remedy for the evils of poisoning the sick because they are sick.

What is needed is a cessation of the practice of poisoning the sick.

CHAPTER XII

The Fallacy of Pharmacology

Medicare (adapted to Psalm 23)
    Medicare is my shepherd; I shall not want.
    It maketh me lie down in bed;
    It leadeth me beside the bottles of pills.
    It restoreth my repugnance to good health.
    Yea, though I walk through the shadow
    Of degenerative diseases, I will feel
    No recrimination or pain;
    For the physician is with me,
    His bedside manners and injections
    Dope and delude me;
    It prepareth me for hell and damnation
    In the presence of "vis meditrix nature";
    It anointeth my hands with antibiotics,
    My blood pressure runneth over.
    Surely weakness and enervation
    Shall follow me all the days of my life;
    And I shall dwell in a heart-lung machine for ever.
    Amen!

> (From "Words & Music and All Alone"
> by K. R. Sidhwa)

Perhaps it is better that the reader understands now why Hygienists consider pharmacology as a pseudo-science. We are not here speaking of the science of chemistry which is incorporated in the basic study of pharmacology, but in the implication therein that pharmacology can interpret correctly the relationship between biology and chemistry.

The Pharmacologist regards man not as a biological being but as a physical entity, that can only react when it is acted upon. All along the Pharmacologists, together with Physiologists, Psychologists, and others have regarded the living organism as capable of acting only when it is acted upon from without. The environment acts upon the body, and then the body reacts.

Hygienists maintain, on the other hand, that a living organism is dynamic and living and full of energy. It maintains itself by the use of this energy, and its self-reparative and restorative ability remains intact as long as the energy is abundant.

Whereas the Pharmacologist believes that the chemical constituents in the living organism organize the life of the organism, the Hygienist believes that the chemical processes and changes are manipulated and organised by this living organism through the energy it possesses.

Dr. Trall supplied the Hygienist answer when he said that in the relations between lifeless matter and the living organism, the living organism is active and the lifeless matter passive. The living organism possesses both the energy of action and the instruments of action.

Applying the principle to drugs, we realise then that it is the body that acts and not the drugs; the drug is not capable of acting either in the human body or without, resting in its bottle.

Pharmacologists, on the other hand, speak about the physiological action of drugs. But such action can only be performed by physiological apparatus, and this only by a living apparatus. Lifeless lungs do not breathe, a lifeless heart does not pulsate, a lifeless stomach does not digest food, and a lifeless nerve fibre transmits no nerve impulses.

Long ago, Samuel Dickson, M.D., wrote in his book "Fallacies of the Faculty" (page 135): "If you divide the pneumo-gastric nerves of a living dog—nerves which as their name imports, connect the brain with the lungs and stomach—arsenic will not produce its accustomed effect on either of these organs". From this it should be obvious to anyone that, if the paralysis of the lungs and stomach by division of the pneumo-gastric nerve, prevented arsenic from "producing" "its accustomed effect" upon these two organs, this is not because the arsenic does not "produce an accustomed effect". It is because the power of action of the lungs and stomach has been destroyed by the operation upon the pneumo-gastric nerve, and not because the power of arsenic to act is destroyed by the operation.

We have said it before, that all foreign substances that enter the body are either inert or poisonous; but apart from the bulk that is in most foodstuffs, the supposedly inert are really poisonous.

The first thing a body does when they are taken in is to make an attempt to organize their removal through the bowels, the skin, the kidneys, the liver, the lungs, the mucous membranes, or by vomiting. This effort is accomplished by rather an uncomfortable and painful process which is termed symptoms.

Foreign materials are either rejected or retained. The resistance and expulsion is a self-preservative effort on the part of the living organism. Sometimes it is very difficult to expel certain chemical substances and may even be dangerous. Then the body adopts another technique for self-preservation—it stores them away in the bones or other tissues for safe keeping—a sort of quarantine. Arsenic, iodine, mercury, bismuth, and common salt are among the materials known to be stored.

When the Pharmacologists talk about a substance as both a toxic substance and a medicinal substance, the two phrases have the same meaning. The poisonous quality of the drugs that produce the vital defensive action of the body is termed the medicinal action of the drug. When drugs are used and side-effects are said to be produced, these side-effects are but some of the disease (discomfort) occasioned by the drug. The so-called physiological and therapeutic effects of these drugs are also disease. If a drug is given to produce a diarrhea, the diarrhea is disease. The laxative action that takes place after taking a purgative is disease.

That drugs are chemical substances, hence capable of Chemical "Action", no one will deny, but the "accustomed effects" of arsenic upon the lungs and stomach are not chemical, else they would not fail to appear when the pneumo-gastric nerve is severed. If these "accustomed effects" were chemical, they would take place after separation of the nerve as readily as before its separation. We refute the assumption that the actions attributed to drugs when taken into the human body are chemical actions. These actions are all together of a different nature from chemical actions. Vomiting, sweating, diarrhea, diuresis, coughing, sneezing, expectoration, redness, swelling narcosis, anaesthesia, etc., are not chemical actions. A blister after a mustard plaster is not formed by chemical action, but as a safeguard against the chemical union of the oil of mustard and flesh. If arsenic combines chemically with flesh, we get arsenate of flesh, and that part of flesh ceases to exist as a physiologically living organism.

The Pharmacologists mistakenly believe that drugs have specific relations to various parts, organs, or structures of the organism, although they have never been able to verify it. Hence began their belief in selective affinity, i.e. certain drugs act on one part of the body, and others act on other parts. That enabled them to classify their drugs into cathartics, emetics, purgatives, diaphoretics, etc. But this is not true as it is often not even possible to tell in advance whether a certain drug shall prove to be an emetic, a purgative, etc. Sometimes on observation one finds that a drug is an emetic, a purgative, etc. If the drugs have the power to perform certain actions, there should be no loss of uniformity in their actions.

The reason their alleged actions are uncertain is because it is the body, the living organism, which chooses the way it is best for them to expel them out of the system. Some drugs will be thrown out of the body via kidney excretion, which the Pharmacologist will call diuretics, another by vomiting, and yet another by expectoration. Some drugs because of their more poisonous nature will be ejected by the body through as many channels as possible, hence its alleged "multiple actions".

Disease is labor, it is struggle. Diseases are exhausting because they are processes of expenditure—they are actions that use up power. For the same reason, drugs are exhausting. If you induce vomiting by means of a physician's drug, it can be using just as much power as vomiting from, say, accidentally eating a fungus.

The body's reservoir of energy or power is not inexhaustible, although the practice of Pharmacologists seems to be based on such a mistaken idea. The more a patient is stimulated (excited, irritated) the weaker he grows, hence, the more drugs, the more danger.

John C. Krantz and C. Jelleff Carr say, in Pharmacologic Principles of Medical Practice (1949), after classifying drugs as stimulants, depressants, irritants, replacements, and bactericides, that, while "most of the agents used in Pharmacology may be classified in one of these five headings", it is certain "that the limits of demarcation among the five classifications are not sharp. There is much overlapping. Further, frequently the character of action refers specifically to one system of the body. Other systems may respond differently to the same drug".

In other words, they are forced unconsciously to assume that the action is really that of the living organism and not that of the drug.

It seems a bit disappointing that after more than a hundred years of intense pharmacological investigation, they have been unable to come up with a more rational explanation of how drugs act, assuming they do, than that contained in the guess that was made over a hundred years ago when Pharmacology was in its infancy, namely, that drugs act on certain parts of the body by virtue of a selective affinity for these parts.

Arthur Gollman in Pharmacology and Therapeutics (1950) says: "The mechanisms of each specific affinity has not been determined; however, the possibility of a specifically directed chemical reaction between the protoplasm of the cells and the drugs which elicit a response is believed to exist".

Thus the whole pharmacological science is based on nothing else but empiriscim. According to the Hygienists the chemical affinities between the constituent of a drug and that of a cell cannot be the cause or the explanation of the action that follows taking drugs. The chemical union of drugs with the constituent of the cells would destroy the cells. It is to prevent this destruction that violent resistive action is taken by the body as a self-preservative action. A blister, for example, is a resistive action to prevent the union of skin cells and oil of mustard. If chemical affinity was the real cause of such an action, it would take place in a dead body, but a dead body does not form a blister when mustard is applied.

In his book "A Textbook of Practical Therapeutics", written way back in 1918, Hobart Amory practically admits the validity of the Hygienist argument. He says that "the recognition of the fact that the body is an aggregation of living cells was shortly followed by the knowledge that, through differentiation and special development, each cell has its own particular function to perform . . . It also became evident that as cells became highly differentiated as to function and form, they became susceptible to influences which failed to affect other special cells, and knowledge of this fact gave impetus to the next step toward modern therapeutics namely, this explained why certain remedies acted upon one part of the body and not on others".

Thus, due to their very constitutional differences, the various structures of the body meet the same emergencies with actions that differ as much as do their normal functions. The lungs can't vomit, neither can the stomach cough, muscle cells do not secrete, and gland cells do not relax and contract. With the understanding of this basic phenomenon, we can now understand why drugs are poisons and Food is food.

The question of where to draw the line never really arises. The Pharmacologists are now getting into a state of panic because they believe that a "witch-hunt" is being directed against them. Because cyclamates, Agene, D.D.T., contraceptive pills, etc. are beiing questioned by governments in the U.S.A. and Britain, the so-called research scientists of the Pharmacological industries are getting worried. The Sunday Telegraph of February 22, 1970, has an article by Gerard Kemp who quotes several research scientists, one of whom said "If everything done on cyclamates was done on every additive, you would end up with no food additives at all, and the problem "How do we feed the population?"

Another important quote comes from Peter Ingham, a Zoologist at Queens University, Belfast, "I question the use of laboratory animals in tests designed to evaluate the probable effect of a chemical on humans. The popular experimental animals—rats, hamsters, guinea pigs—are the products of intensive and deliberate inbreeding. "This is advantageous to the 'pure' researcher studying normal physiology, but tends to produce a weaker strain of animal with less natural resistance.

"The laboratory animal might well be expected to show adverse responses to abnormal chemical and physical conditions, which might have no effect on its hardier wild counterpart".

Thank you, Mr. Ingham—you have answered very clearly the question that many people have asked the Hygienists—"Why is it that only some people show adverse effects on taking drugs and others don't seem to?" Man is a tougher and more complex organism and not so easy to destroy, and some constitutions require more abuse than others before they eventually succumb. Besides, as we have emphasized before, the relationship of one kind of species with a poison varies with that of another. In final effort man is the only true guinea pig for any experimentation, and short term experiments of a few months or years are not sufficient. One needs a generation or two to notice the accumulated effects of all the abuse piled upon man.

No doubt, when speaking before the Delhi Medical Association, C. E. Paget, M.D., a noted British Pharmacologist, had this to say in The Statesman, New Delhi, February 1, 1967, in an address on "Withdrawal of Drugs from Medical Practice."

"That not only are modern drugs wrongly used, but their pharmacology, clinical, and statistical trials are too short to study their dangerous potentialities."

He added that if a balance sheet of the risks and benefits of modern drugs was drawn up, the risks would certainly be found to be bigger. And rightly so, because the drug-induced diseases have been largely of the chronic variety and have proved very difficult to remedy in a radical way. These diseases range from skin rashes and ashthma to hepatitis, aplastic anemia, leukemia, and even cancer. Cases of cataract with blindness, spontaneous breaking of bones, and deafness have resulted from some of the new drugs.

As this is written, we find that the picture painted by us of the medicated society of today is truly confirmed in two books which have just come to our attention. One is "The Medicated Society" edited by Samuel Proger, M.D. The other is "The Coming Revolution in Medicine" by David D. Rutstein, M.D.

An excerpt from the former states very clearly what is meant by a medicated society: "The American public is said to be drug-happy, using enormous quantities of prescription drugs along with self-prescribed medicines ranging from aspirin and antacids to tranquilizers, rubbing compounds, and suppositories. Approximately one billion prescriptions are filled annually in this country—that is double the number that were filled just ten years ago and represents about five prescriptions for every man, woman and child . . . Then there are the non-prescription drugs . . .

More than half of the drug purchases comes from over the counter . . . People seem to have become more disease-conscious, and they seek medical aid for more trifling ailments, or they take drugs for no ailment at all."

It is true to say that the modern day society is fast arriving at the stage where it is taken for granted that no one can possibly live out his or her life without the support of medicine. Drugs and medicines have spilled over into other departments of human life, from the passing of examinations to achievements in sports and games.

The statement from the latter book, however, goes to show that all this effort of being "a medicated society" has been in vain and all the research fruitless and full of delusions.

Dr. Rutstein says that "this enormous expansion in our national medical research program, together with our lagging national health picture, is the paradox of modern medicine." He goes on to say, with regards to life expectancy, "during the past two decades, the lengthening of life expectancy has ground almost to a halt. Indeed, we have failed to keep up with the improved life expectancy in many other countries, and the trend has worsened in the last several years." During the past two or three decades, the improvement in our infant mortality rate has slowed down."

This paradox, we have shown, is not due to lack of money or effort on the part of the medical researcher, but to the fact that medicine and its system of drug pushing is self-perpetuating in the sense that it does not eradicate or "cure" disease, but merely changes its pattern and adds to the complications and side-effects, which we are now told are responsible for ten percent of hospital admissions.

In matters of health, we Hygienists feel that there is too much reliance on an elite that is supposed to fix the world. The medical profession, like any other elite group, gets professionalized and forgets about the problem they're trying to fix—namely, abundant health for the people—and ends up with palliation of symptoms. We do not admit that the medical profession has all the answers to human health and welfare. We reject the notion that medical experts are best qualified to deal with social and psychological questions in relationship with health and wholesomeness. In fact, often it is just the opposite. Children learn more from other children than from teachers; poor people may be better qualified to deal with poverty problems than social workers; prisonsers know more about crime prevention than criminologists; mental patients are often more helpful to each other than the psychiatric staff; and people who have studied health, i.e. Hygienists, Food-Reformers, and Nature cure people more than medical scientists who study disease and all its pathology. "If the doors of perception were cleansed, every thing would appear to man as it is, infinite," wrote Blake. "For man has closed himself up, till he sees all things through narrow chunks of his cavern."

To those like the medical profession who have made pharmacology their God, the infinite moment of intuitive perception can be interpreted either negatively or positively. It is either an escape or an entrance, either self-extinction or re-birth. It is self-extinction for those who believe that Pharmacology and Health are synonymous. For those who use it as a beginning to newer concepts of health, it is a re-birth.

And in medicine as in agriculture, the need for a new attitude to germs and viruses is becoming urgent. The accepted cycle—resistant strain, new drugs, high pressure salesmanship, extensive use, resistant strain—is highly profitable to the Pharmaceutical Industries.

If there were no resistant strains, the industry would fold up. But this cycle is not only dangerous but expensive to the community. Not only does it perpetuate the life cycle of germs, but also the fear that such an approach encourages. When the medical profession changes its attitude and realises that the need is not to concentrate on ways to destroy hostile "disease agents" but to find why they became hostile in order to learn how to convert them into pacific ways again, only then will the social hazards of Pharmacology be minimized.

One of the greatest social hazards involved is to make the society as a whole dependent on drugs .The pharmaceutical industry, however, justifies its existence and that of chemotherapy by wrongly attributing the effect on the life span in civilized countries to the use of drugs.

Even if this was true, and it is not, longevity is a poor measure of the health of a community; and there is enough data to prove that in many respects people in civilized countries have been getting progressively unhealthier, and that a great deal of responsibility for this could be attributed to medical treatments.

Even Dr. Herbert Ratner, Professor in a Chicago medical school and Commissioner of Health in the state of Illinois, U.S.A., berates about this in a most forthright manner, while admitting that the United States has become the most over-medicated, most over-operated, most over-inoculated country in the world, as well as the most anxiety-ridden in regard to health and disease. He says, "We are flabby, overweight, and have a lot of dental caries, fluoridation notwithstanding. Our gastrointestinal system operates like a spluttering gas engine. We can't sleep; we can't get going when we are awake. We have neuroses. We have high blood pressure. Neither our hearts nor our heads last as long as they should. Coronary disease at the peak of life has hit epidemic proportions. Suicide is one of the leading causes of death, fourth, between the ages of of fifteen and forty-four. We suffer from a plethora of the disease of civilization."

He continues: "We have become increasingly a paying animal, as if health was solely a commodity of the market place. Barbiturates, stimulants, and tranquilizers have been the most misused. We consume fantastic amounts of these drugs. For many they are used as a panacea to solve personal problems. They are practically replacing the functions of the virtues in striving for a sane and well-ordered life . . . We are becoming a pill-swallowing civilization, and God help us as a nation and as individuals when the new contraceptive pill really gets going."

Previous to this outburst by Dr. Ratner, Dr. William Evans, consulting physician to the Cardiac Department of the London Hospital, expressed a similar point of view about Britain in September, 1962, when he admitted that the expenditure on drugs had doubled here in the course of eight years. He rightly inquired whether it meant that more lives had been saved, or health recaptured, at a corresponding rate, or did it simply mean that the nation was being doped? The doctor was in no doubt; the huge number of prescriptions and a corresponding increase in the kind of drugs was "evidence of the unquenchable thirst for mixtures and potions, and the unsatiable appetite for pills and tablets, exhibited by the public. Credulity in the power of medicines to do good knows no bounds. Such confirmed addiction by the "philophysic", a product of twentieth century expansion of the drug industry, though largely self-inflicted, has been contracted with the connivance of the medical profession, which has remained wholly passive as the contagious affliction spreads."

So the pharmaceutical industry has succeeded in what it has consciously or unconsciously set out to do. It has made us all, in one way or other, addicted to drugs, and all the signs are that this dependence is still growing.

The fallacy of pharmacology is thus perpetuated into the heart and minds of the population as a whole, as well as the earnest and eager medical student of the future. What is needed most is to tell these young students that drugs are palliatives and basically symptom removers. The next step is to bring to their attention the study of the basic causes of disease. But we cannot expect the pharmaceutical industry to finance such a venture; and the medical profession, in spite of the efforts of individuals, is too fossilised to change its outlook rapidly and quickly. The teaching of a healthy way of life is too important a subject to be left to the doctors—not because they are less intelligent or trustworthy than other people, but simply because they suffer from the usual symptoms of a trade union kind of monopoly—proneness to self-opinionated bureaucracy— inability to learn from others, inclination to go on not merely accepting but teaching false principles they were taught years ago, even though irrelevant to the study of health; and finally because they do not want to admit that the whole edifice of medicine and pharmacology is based on empirical concepts.

However, we do not agree with other writers (e.g. Brian Inglis in Drugs, Doctors and Disease) when they say that the public is to blame for this sort of situation. The public, the mass, the media, are like sheep—they follow—and what is easier to follow than the concept that health can be bought from a bottle and without any effort on the part of the individual to discipline his day-to-day life? Once such an idea was formulated and the industry was launched, it became very difficult for most medical physicians to re-trench from that viewpoint.

Both the medical profession and the public are to be blamed for suffering from what Edmond Cahn described as the Pharaoh syndrome, and the Pompey syndrome, at the Johns Hopkins Conference.

When Pharaoh built a pyramid, he presumably considered the hundreds of thousands of human lives lost as part of the overall expense; they were expendable. Both the public and the medical profession have allowed themselves to be lulled by such phrases as "the social cost of progress" into accepting the so-called "side-effects" and hazards of chemotherapy as "natural and inevitable," forgetting that the personal cost in lives, deformities, pain, and distress may actually outweigh the benefits of palliating symptoms.

When Pompey's lieutenant suggested that they should murder his guests, Antony and Caesar, Pompey replied:

"Ah, this thou should'st have done
And not have spoken out! In me 'tis villainy
In thee't had been good service."

In the words of Edmond Cahn: "We have the most pervasive of moral syndromes, the most characteristic of so-called respectable men in a civilized society. To possess the end and yet not be responsible for the means, to grasp the fruit while still disavowing the tree, to escape being told the cost until somebody else has paid it irrevocably—this is the Pompey syndrome, and the chief hypocrisy of our time. In the days of the outcry against Thalidomide, how much of popular indignation might be attributed to this same syndrome! How many were furious because their own lack of scruple had been exposed!

"So many did not really care, did not even want to know what the new drugs might cost in terms of human injuries and fatalities. The dispensers of Thalidomide had outraged the public by breaking an unwritten law—the law against interrupting the public's enjoyment of fruits, with disagreeable revelations about the tree and the soil where the fruits have grown."

But Edmond Cahn cannot have it both ways, as most physicians want to have. Who nurtured the idea into the public image that drugs are safe and that taking them brings health? Who but the medical profession have taught the public to believe that drugs are only dangerous when self-prescribed and not when prescribed by a physician? If it is not the physicians, who else then has taught the public to believe that looking after people's welfare in matters of health and disease be left alone to the "specialists" who know what they are doing? If it is not the pharmaceutical industry, who else, with the connivance of the medical profession, tried to hide from the public and play down the news of the Thalidomide tragedy and suggestions that deformities may be caused by the administration of antibiotics during pregnancy, for fear the news would worry pregnant mothers and upset the whole faith of the world at large in drugs and medicines?

It is absurd for physicians to claim that they have a right to prescribe whatever drug they feel is best for the patient because they alone are qualified to do so, when the whole history of pharmaceuticals rebuts that claim. At the same time and in the same breath they claim it is the duty of the public to be aware of any misdemeanors—how can this be so?

It is obvious that as long as the medical profession with its belief centered in Pharmacology is permitted to enjoy the monopoly that it now has, to control its own education and its prescribing privileges, it is hard to see how it can be brought back to a realisation of its true responsibilities and vocation of teaching people the art of healthy living.

CHAPTER XIII

Drugs and Chemicals in Our Food and Drinks

The public buys its opinions as it buys its milk, on the principle that it is cheaper to do this than to keep a cow. So it is, but the milk is more likely to be watered —Samuel Butler

The appalling shortage of scientists probably explains why certain kinds of food are still eatable—Beachcomber (Daily Express 24/4/59)

Many people would be aghast if they were told to consume a pinch of arsenic or belladonna, or a drop of prussic acid or potassium hydrocyanide. They would be frightened to touch it even, in case they should accidentally injure or kill themselves. Yet in millions of homes people are slowly but surely sending themselves to an early grave because of their unconscious addiction to one form of "poison" or another in the ordinary, everyday things they take into their bodies.

Madam, if tea is your favorite beverage, then it is time you knew something about its contents. Tea contains caffeine and theophylline, as well as large amounts of tannic acid. It is less harmful than ordinary coffee, but its effects are more lasting. A consumption of 30 cups a day—and, believe it or not, people do drink such quantities—produces depression of breathing and hallucinations. Those who are not used to strong tea can have convulsions after from three to five cups. So much for those who say, "I like my brew dark and strong." It can cause derangement of the nervous system, headaches, loss of memory, disorders of vision and shrinking of the liver, as well as trembling, palpitations, restlessness and kidney troubles. If you are fond of yerba mate tea, you should know that this also

153

contains caffeine, and although the amount is less than in ordinary tea, it is very habit-forming.

If you are a coffee-pot addict, then you too are not out of the wood. Ordinary coffee not only contains caffeine but other alkaloids as well, notably theobromine. Too frequent coffee-breaks can lead to coffee-breakdown, some of the symptoms of which are garrulousness and restlessness, cardiac pains, loss of appetite, nausea, insomnia, and headaches.

In an article in "Science Today", August 1966, Mr. Irwin Ross lists the "startling things" that happen inside the human organism when one or two cups of coffee are taken. This is what he says: "Within a few minutes the temperature of your stomach jumps 10 to 15 degrees F., and there is an increase of up to 400 percent in its secretion of hydrochloric acid. Your salivary glands double their output; your heart beats 15 per cent harder. Blood vessels get narrower in and around your heart. Your metabolic rate goes up by 25 percent, your kidneys excrete 100 percent more urine." Apart from that, coffee drinking leads to hypoglycemia, which is the opposite of diabetes, and eventual breakdown of the pancreatic system. Do you still want a coffee-break?

In his "Textbook of Pharmacology", Professor W. T. Salter says this about tea and coffee: "The chief problem with methylxanthine beverages (tea and coffee) . . . is the possible chronic effect on the central nervous system. Excessive and prolonged use . . . clearly may lead to increased irritability, loss of sleep, palpitation of the heart, and even muscular tremors. Such effects are due to chronic mild intoxication with caffeine and other alkaloids found in both tea and coffee." You have been warned!

The cola drinks which are now so fashionable with children and adolescents contain caffeine and phosphoric acid, and their regular consumption can make caffeine addicts of your children as well as cause their teeth to decay.

If, on the other hand, you are a chocolate and cocoa fan, then you may not be aware that cocoa, from which of course chocolate is made, contains both caffeine and theobromine, and so, as in the case of coffee, rapid pulse, headaches and trembling can result from its excessive consumption.

If tobacco is your favorite poison, then you should know that there is no more virulent substance than nicotine. Only prussic acid is comparable with it. A drop of pure nicotine held before the beak of a bird will kill it. Heavy smokers can absorb 20 mg. of nicotine in an hour. In the case of the novice smoker, nicotine first irritates, and then finally paralyses some of the cells of the vegetative nervous system, giving rise to nausea, pallor, cold sweats, giddiness, retching, lassitude, and limpness, which may last for hours after the first cigarette has been smoked. On the other hand, the 20-a-day smoker may suffer headaches, dizziness, palpitations, and stabbing pains in the heart and left arm, shortness of breath, and a sense of chilliness. Nerve pains and neuralgia tend to become increasingly intense, and disorders of vision develop and may persist. Red-rimmed "tobacco eyes", "smoker's cough", chronic pharyngitis, intractible insomnia, and lung cancer complete the picture of the effects of cigarette smoking.

Those who cannot eat a meal without a liberal dressing of salt should be told that inorganic sodium chloride is a virulent poison for the living organism. From 1 to 3 grams of salt can cause a condition known as salt fever in infants. In adults, besides inducing kidney breakdown, hypertension and the retention of fluid in the tissues (edema), the excessive consumption of salt may lead to various kinds of skin inflammation, dry, cracked skin, profuse sweating, falling hair, dry scalp, nerve pain, headaches, eye pains, and attacks of giddiness. The mucous membranes may become inflamed, leading to colds, gastro-intestinal catarrh, diarrea and gingivitis and in pregnant mothers, to a condition known as eclampsia of pregnancy.

As early as 1900 it was shown by Linossier that the amount of salt consumed at an ordinary meal retarded protein digestion to the same extent as would a reduction of from 40 to 50 percent in the amount of pepsin—one of the gastric juices secreted by the stomach. A further explanation of the digestive impairment which salt induces is that by disguising the flavor of foods, it hinders the exact adaption of the digestive juices to the particular food that is being eaten.

The relation of salt to insomnia and nervous ailments has been studied by Dr. Mickail M. Miller, of the U.S.A. He found that insomnia could be reduced in direct proportion to the rate at which he withheld salt from the diet. Also, many sufferers from Meniere's disease (a common cause of giddiness) improved and eventually recovered completely when salt was eliminated from their diet, which previously had contained salt in large quantities.

Alcohol is another very popular poison. In fact, it seems that we are not only a well-preserved but a well-pickled nation if we can judge from the many alcoholics and social drinkers we have in the country. It takes one hour for the body to burn up 7 grams of alcohol, which means 1¼ hours for an average glass of spirit or wine. An intake of 250 grams of alcohol can be fatal—and a bottle of whiskey contains this amount. Exercise does not help the body to burn up alcohol as it does other high-calorie commodities.

Recently a life insurance company quoted the death rate of "regular spirit drinkers" as being 83 percent higher than that of total abstainers. The ill effects of alcohol upon the human system are already common knowledge, and little needs to be added here, apart from saying that modern physiological studies have confirmed the frequent assertions made by temperance workers that it harms the heart, blood vessels and nerves, as well as other organs. There is absolutely no truth in the popular belief that alcohol aids digestion or contributes in any way to good health.

To this list of some common social poisons we might add the newer and as yet less common substances such as the various psychedelic drugs, including LSD, which apart from being habit-forming, are a danger to the life and sanity of the individual.

All habits start from very small beginnings. There are many incentives—good health, happiness, financial savings —for replacing poison habits with good habits, such as eating good quality wholesome food, taking plenty of fresh air, exercise, rest, relaxation, etc. Why not make a start now?

However, these are things which people take knowingly into their bodies, but many people do not realize that drugs are spilled over in our various food and drink in more ways than one.

It is now being gradually realised that our environment is being polluted. Our air is full of chemical fumes, our water polluted through drugs and sewage waste from chemical factories, threatening not only the lives of those that live in the sea but humans also—added to it the medically foisted idea of having to add sodium fluoride in our drinking water—a poison if ever there was one. Even the chlorination of our public water supplies may not be the innocent thing that it appears to be. Chlorine and other chlorine compounds are powerful oxidising and bleaching agents. When the chlorination of water produces an offensive taste and smell, enough chlorine may enter the intestinal tract to destroy bacteria and thus deprive us of the essential vitamins which they make for us. Fluorides are strong inhibitors of enzymes, especially those concerned with the utilization of sugars and starches. Our soil is being polluted by chemical fertilizers, and the crops on such depleted soil when disease-ridden is sprayed with insecticides and pesticides to be given to us as food. One has only to read the late Rachel Carson's book "Silent Spring" to realize the dangers and the tragic-comic battle which the insecticide industry wages with the insect world—a battle which the insects are clearly winning—but which we as human beings are slowly losing in that we are slowly but surely killing ourselves with poisons from our own backyard.

But this is the age of the "calculated risk". This means different things to different people. The public, who usually have to take the risk, are constantly being reassured that when "calculated", a given risk is negligible. To those creating the peril, it means, "The odds are we can get away with it."

Unfortunately our present culture is dominated by a simple-minded test-tube approach to biology. The laws of biology, however, are intricate. All living beings on this earth exist in a system governed by an incredibly sensitive complex of checks and balances. We can learn these laws of nature and adapt them to our needs, or we can defy them and perish.

If we come to our senses tomorrow, the damage accomplished in a single decade will take generations to undo. If, however, we continue our present deadly progress, there is no telling what the consquences will be.

With the coming of the industrial revolution, technology began to take over our civilization and today, because it can control all the steps in a manufacturing process, we have come to believe that medicine and agriculture can use technology to exercise a similar control over disease and food production.

But the "cure" and prevention of disease is not just a

matter of technology. It is actually applied biology. Like agriculture, it too must deal with living things living off other living things. Soil management is a matter of applied biology. If man is to reach the goal of perfect health, or even continue to have it as an objective, agriculture must be re-directed toward an appreciation of the biological inter-relationship that exists between every living thing, especially in the soil, and redirected away from the chemical test tube. Sir Albert Howard's "Agricultural Testament" should be available as a textbook to all students of agriculture.

What most of us fail to appreciate, perhaps because it seems to be beyond our comprehension, is that the enzymatic processes in our bodies are affected even by slight traces of chemicals—by as little as one part in fifty million or less. The possibility of harmful effects of a slowly accumulative nature in dilutions is a new discovery. The effects cannot yet be measured by analytical methods—hence the turning of blind-eye attitude of those that be in power when it comes to meddling with our food and drink.

The recent ban on cyclamates in America, Britain, and other countries is a case in point. Facts are we do not know all the facts, and it may take 40 years or more, but meanwhile the damage will have been done. The benefit of any doubt should be given to living things—people, animals, plants, etc. and not to chemical industries. Our motto should be "if in doubt—cut it out."

Many millions of people are half sick as a result of chemicals added to their food. These chemicals inhibit the enzymatic actions which are so essential to healthy living. The chemicals, among other things, can produce a vitamin deficiency, even though the person may be eating what is generally called a balanced diet. Dr. Jonathan Forman, M.D., an enlightened physician, says: "The vitamins which we emphasize as essential to health are constantly destroyed for us in the following ways.

(1) By oxidation in storage and in cooking. By sterilizing and other forms of processing. (2) Many supposedly harmless drugs, some containing lead, mercury, arsenic and bismuth, interrupt enzymatic reactions and hence are strong antagonists. These minerals not only inhibit the action of enzymes by displacing the mineral-catalyzing portions of

the enzyme, they also greatly increase excretion of vitamins in the urine. (3) Most astringents, laxatives, and solvents seriously deplete the tissues of their vitamin content. (4) Narcotics and pain-killers such as nicotine, alcohol, morphine, barbiturates, and aspirin are well recognised vitamin antagonists consumed in great excess by our people. (5) Antibiotics in a considerable degree owe their effectiveness to their destruction of bacteria in the alimentary canal. This means either the death of favorable bacteria which manufacture essential vitamins, or the overgrowth of the unfriendly bacteria which prevent the growth of these helpful bacteria. At the same time these unfriendly bacteria may even produce toxins themselves. (6) Bleaching agents, such as agene, formerly used in baking bread, chlorine dioxide now used in its place, benzoyl peroxide, or alkaline persulphate have a very strong tendency to destroy most vitamins, but especially the oil soluble Vitamins A, D, E and K. The extent to which bleaching agents of one sort or another are used to bleach common foods is little appreciated by those of us not in the food industry. (7) Sulphuring of foods for preservation, as in the preparation of dried fruits such as raisins, prunes, apricots, peaches, and apples. To this list must be added the sulphides which are employed to "freshen" meats and give them a better color.

So you think you know what you are eating? Additives you have never even heard of come as part of every commercial food you buy. Some time ago, 1965-66, Lady Dartmouth told an audience at the National Institute of Nutrition a story describing a housewife's typical shopping expedition. "She starts at the butcher's. 'I'll have a nice cut of beef', she says. She doesn't know that the animal has been given tranquilizers. Then from the fishmonger she buys some cod. She doesn't know that in the trawler it has been preserved in ice impregnated with antibiotics. Then to the dairy. She needs extra milk as her children have friends to tea. She doesn't know that 11 percent of the milk in England and Wales contains penicillin injected directly into cows' udders to prevent mastitis, and that published evidence shows that penicillin in milk gives humans dermatitis and urticaria, a nasty, scratchy disease."

The food you eat now is definitely not the same that

reached the tables of your forefathers. Food has never been so processed, added to, and impregnated with chemicals and coloring matter as it is today. There are over 3,000 chemicals added to our commercialised food items in one way or other.

From the London Sunday Express of February 17, 1963, we get a story of how an owner of a Scottish mink herd was awarded over $20,000 by an Edinburgh Court because a firm sent him capon offal as food for his mink. Capons are young neutered cocks injected with drugs (antibiotics and hormones) to fatten them; but after feeding on the offal, the mink became as sterile as the cocks. Can you imagine a person with an eye for a fast buck selling capon offal to humans instead of the pill? It is not as far fetched as you think; some people just have no principles.

We need another Dr. Harvey W. Wiley, a champion of pure food if ever there was one. Because Theodore Roosevelt made the Pure Food and Drug Act a law in 1906 by placing his signature on it, he is given the credit for originating it also. The credit, however, belongs to Wiley and his band of dedicated assistants who fought big business even then to prevent food adulteration.

He helped to put a ban on many of the coal tar dyes, the adding of saccharine, and various other things. However, Big Business was far too big for Wiley and gradually it took over, so that once again we are eating "chemical junk" rather than food.

The chief danger from manufactured food is that it may contain chemicals which would not normally be consumed in this manner. A perfect example is provided by white bread, which undergoes treatment with chemical "improvers", emulsifiers, anti-staling agents, and bleaches, among other things, and by the time it reaches our plates it contains virtually no natural vitamins or other nutritional properties, except "Pure starch"; it is in fact a toxic substance, all the former goodness having been obliterated in the milling and manufacturing process.

In his book, "Cancer: Nature, Cause and Cure", Dr. Alexander Berglas said that the incidence of cancer in civilized races (one out of four will contract the disease) was due largely to the noxious agents deliberately placed on, around and in us, and for this the wholesale adulteration of food is largely to blame.

That D.D.T. is now being banned in various countries is a good thing as it is now being shown that it has very lethal effects, and the body finds it very hard to eliminate it from the system. Writing in the November 1975 issue of "Health for All", a British periodical on health and allied matters, the writer, Edgar York, comments very strongly about the D.D.T. now being found in mothers' milk.

We know that good normal breast milk is the best food for babies, and Hygienists and other nutritionists have claimed that it is better than cows' milk. We do not yet know just what damage its contamination by D.D.T. may do, nor do we know the vital fact as to whether any such damage outweighs the known benefits of breast feeding. Until we have reliable data on this point I believe that breast feeding should continue, and that mothers should do their utmost to get organically-grown fruits, vegetables and cereals. They should also press the Government to forbid the use of these dangerous chemicals in agriculture so as to reduce the contamination of breast milk.

Mr. York's article is such an eye-opener that I am quoting it in full to show how chemicals contaminate our children's lives from the moment they are born.

'Precious Poison'

In an article in the French magazine "Nature et Progrès", towards the end of 1974, Claude Aubert wrote that mother's milk—'the most precious and irreplaceable of all foods'—has become the most toxic. Four years ago, in the same magazine, Aubert reported that nursing babies in Sweden imbibe from their mother's milk three to four times more DDT than the limit set for foodsuffs by the World Health Organisation. An investigation carried out by the Milk Industries Laboratory in Douai, in collaboration with 10 'mother's milk stations' in various French towns, revealed that the situation in France is now similar to, if not worse than, the situation in Sweden four years ago. The breast-fed baby—man at the most sensitive stage of his life—receives almost exclusively the food that is most polluted with toxic residues. In the tests, which extended from November 1972 to October 1973, 250 to 500-gramme samples of milk from mothers in Bordeaux, Lyons, Nantes, St. Etienne, Lille, Marmande, Rouen and Strasbourg were examined monthly for toxic residues. The milk was collected from 30 to 40 mothers in each town and analyzed for residues of the main pesticides of the chlorinated hydrocarbon group—i.e. HCH, HCB, aldrin, dieldrin, heptachlor, epoxyde, DDT and their derivatives. In other words, the investigations covered only *one* aspect of the general toxic situation; the newer organic phosphorus compounds were not included.

" *'Alarming Results'*

The values determined for the individual towns are the mean from 12-monthly samples, collected from each of the 30-40 mothers—i.e. the average of approximately four hundred test samples. The mean figure for France is thus the average of 4,000 test samples from 350 mothers. The highest figures for HCH and HCB were reached in St. Etienne, where mother's milk contained 3.53 parts per thousand (p.p.t.) while in Paris the value was 2.75 p.p.t. The mean value for the whole country was 2.75 p.p.t., whereas the average figure for cow's milk is only 0.18 p.p.t. Residues from aldrin and dieldrin were highest in Marmande, with a figure of 0.28 mg per kg (Paris 0.24 mg) while the national value was 0.23 mg. The national figure for cow's milk was 0.05 mg. The results could be summarized as follows:

1)   Mother's milk in France is significantly more toxic than cow's milk, containing 16 times more HCH and HCB and five times more aldrin and dieldrin.

2)   The toxic residues are several times higher than the tolerances permitted by the World Health Organisation for milk products. Mother's milk contains five and a half times more HCH and HCB and twice as much aldrin and dieldrin as the permitted amounts.

3)   The level of toxicity in the whole of France is very high. There is no significant difference between the north and south, nor between town and country.

" Nevertheless, protests that immoderate amounts of organic chlorides are being used are inevitably countered by official statements that, in this particular field, French law is the strictest in the world, and that the safety measures in force are such that the danger of poisoning is reduced virtually to nil. The results of the investigations reveal that all the allegedly stringent security measures have had little effect, since the level of toxicity of French mother's milk is higher than that in all other countries, except that the DDT content is higher in Germany. 'Nature et Progrès' examined the situation under two headings:

How can the results be explained? It is quite feasible that household insecticides could be contributing to the poisoning of mother's milk, but it is incontestable that food is the main source of poisoning. This opinion is shared by M. Luquet, director of the Milk Industries' Laboratory, who led the investigations. Proof was provided by the fact that milk from mothers who used no insecticides in the home contained an equally high amount of toxic residues. The reason why the toxic residues in mother's milk are considerably greater than in cow's milk is that the residues have accumulated in the fatty tissues over the years, and can only be discharged via the milk.

Consequences for babies' health. None of the responsible authorities can or will give information on this problem. Apparently, no one knows whether the residues are dangerous for babies. There are, however, several astonishing facts:

1)   It has been known for several years that mother's milk contains toxic residues, and that in other countries also mother's milk is more toxic than cow's milk—but nothing has been done.

2)   As soon as the level of toxicity was known, the following measures should have been introduced: a) Investigation of the state of health and development of babies in relation to their nutrition and the residue-content of the mother's milk, and comparisons wih those children receiving an artificial diet; b) Investigations into the health of animals whose young are given milk with various degrees of residual pollution.

"   According to Aubert, no such tests have been carried out. Nevertheless, it is a fact that a three-month-old breast-fed baby receiving 900 grams of milk daily ingests four times more DDT, four times more heptachlor and seven times more dieldrin than the tolerance limits set down by the World Health Organisation. Moreover, these are mean values which are probably considerably exceeded in some individual cases.

"   *'What can be Done?'*

As soon as the results of the investigations were known,

it was important to examine the position of mothers who endeavour to eat only natural, organically-grown produce and who, as can be expected, also strive, as far as possible, to breast-feed their babies. Several mothers among the readers of 'Nature et Progres' were willing to allow their milk to be analysed and to fill in a questionnaire containing 16 questions concerning their eating habits. These questions sought to establish the type of nutrition and the source of the food, whereby a distinction could be made between bought mass-produced food, bought organically-grown food, and self-grown organic produce. Furthermore, possible changes in the diet and the sources of produce in recent years were also investigated, and the mothers were also asked whether household insecticides were in use.

" As experience has shown that not all products designated 'organic' fully deserve the title, such bought products were valued as only 40 to 50 percent organic but, nevertheless, the results proved to be consistent.

" 'Results of the Investigation'

In spite of the relatively small number (16) of mothers who took part in the test, the information obtained was illuminating:

1) There is a definite relationship between the level of toxic residues in the mother's milk and the amount of organically grown produce in the diet. The greater the proportion of organic food, the less the amount of toxic residues.

2) Compared with the average figures for other French mothers, the milk of mothers eating 70 to 80 percent organically grown food contained on average only 40 percent of the HCH and HCB, 50 percent of the heptachlor and 37 percent of the DDT and its derivatives.

" It is therefore essential that when a natural diet is consumed, consisting mainly of whole cereal products, vegetables and fruits, the foodstuffs should be organically grown without the use of pesticides. The French tests showed that in families in which mainly whole cereals are consumed, and which are not organically grown, or in which less than 50 percent are organically grown, the mother's milk is more polluted than that of the average French mother. This is a matter of vital importance to food-reformers, particularly vegetarian food-reformers. The

term 'organically-grown' is, of course, understood to mean
also free from pesticides.
"   Dr. Hans Heinze, Germany's pioneer of bio-dynamic
agriculture, who published the French report in the journal
'Lebendige Erde', appended the following conclusions:
1)   Our protests against the use of pesticides are more
than justified, even—or especially—when we are assured
that all safety measures have been taken.
2)   The prohibition of chlorinated hydrocarbons (DDT,
etc.) does little to solve the problem, since the confirmed
dangers of these present products will be confirmed again
in 10 to 20 years time with regard to the organic phosphorus compounds and herbicides, doubtless not in the
form of residues, but probably in the form of other chemical problems—less visible, but all the more serious.
3)   It is all the more necessary to be unyielding in oppos-
ing the use of chemical herbicides and pesticides in any
form.
4)   Biological agriculture, which has proved its efficiency
and success over decades, is the only long-term solution to
our agrarian problems.
5)   Consumers who wish to obtain organically-grown
produce should compel the suppliers to provide a guarantee
as to the authenticity of their wares.
"   Further evidence of the urgency of the pesticide problem was provided by Professor Hans Holtmeier in the German medical magazine, 'Deutsches Artzeblatt'.
"   'Insufficiently Researched'
    The most alarming factor, according to Holtmeier, is
the increasing pollution of mother's milk due to the storing
of these toxic chemicals in the fatty tissues. As far back
as 1973, an analysis of the milk from German mothers had
given values up to twenty times greater than the permitted
tolerance level for ordinary foodstuffs. A baby could thus
ingest from his mother's milk up to twice the quantity of
these substances that is permitted for long-term nutrition.
Even three-month-old embryos and five-day-old babies had
an 'alarming' amount of these noxious chemicals in their
fatty tissues. Even now, little is known of the long-term
effects of chemical pesticides on human tissue. According
to Holtmeier, there are roughly 1,600 different types of
pesticides in common use.

"   In a recently-published table, mother's milk in the USA in 1969 contained the comparatively low level of 0.02 mg per kg of DDT and its derivatives but, in the intervening seven years, the quantity has probably increased considerably. In the same period the figures for Holland have jumped from 0.05 to 2.5 mg per kg, exceeded only by France (3.2) and Germany (3.8). Unfortunately I have no figures for Britain, but perhaps Margaret Brady could give readers more information on this topic which is of particular importance to families endeavouring to follow a natural way of life.   "

Moreover, in a conference in London in August/September 1975 it was also pointed out that pain-killing drugs taken by mothers of breast-fed babies slowed up the baby's reflexes and thus interfered with normal breast-feeding.

Cyclamate, an artificial sweetner, was banned in the USA and Britain only in 1969. Yet in December 1967, an article entitled "Artificial Sweeteners a Menace to Health" by the author of this book, appeared in "Health for All", a British publication. That use of cyclamates may result in the birth of deformed offspring (another Thalidomide disaster) or the pre-birth death of babies is not a far-fetched thought. Experiments have shown that cyclamate not only curbed the growth of test animals, but also stunted the growth of their young. Other possible side-effects indicated by experiments were mental retardation, body rashes, dizziness, diarrhoea, and itching. Soft drinks are no more, no less than just coloured poison. Our children consume it from their babyhood, and yet we sit back and let them be slowly poisoned. In America in 1960, 10 million cases of cyclamate-containing drinks were consumed, and by 1967 the total had zoomed to over 400 million cases. Can you now imagine how the manufacturers must have fought bitterly to stop it from being banned, and why it took so many years for the governments of the U.S.A. and Britain to come to a decision to stop it? The stink was very big, and it just could not be hidden any longer, but it was a battle every inch of the way.

The same thing happened when Rachel Carson's book "Silent Spring" came out in 1962 in the U.S.A. Before it was published a year later in Britain, the Association of

Agricultural Chemical Manufacturers sent an expensively printed brochure to every likely reviewer. It criticized the book's "emotional attitude", ignored the 61 pages of scientific references supporting the author's frightening attack on modern pesticides and included carefully worded passages, damning the book with faint praise, which would be suitable for inclusion in a "review" by lazy journalists.

On January 1, 1970, more than five years after her book, Sweden became the first country to enforce a complete ban on the organo-chlorine compounds (D.D.T. being the best known).

Once upon a time . . . a glass of orange juice was simply juice from an orange; butter was churned mlik, nothing more; a piece of meat had nothing in it but the spices *you* added in cooking it. If you wanted to take your chances on a piece of chocolate cake, a look at the recipe would tell you the whole story of how much sugar and white flour your body would have to contend with—there would be no unknown ingredient in the flour or the chocolate. Even with ice cream or candy you knew what you were up against, and if you wanted to eat such things . . . well, the risk was yours. Today, if you want to eat these things, the risk is still yours, but with this difference: to understand just what you're up against, you'd have to be a chemical engineer!

Food additives have become a mighty part of the food industry in the past 35 years. It is almost impossible to purchase a commercially produced food product that has not been treated in some way to give it a characteristic the producer wants it to have, or one he's educated the consumer to want and expect. There are hardeners and softeners, foaming agents and anti-foaming agents, acidifiers, and alkalizers, bleaches, coloring agents, thickeners, and so on—ad nauseum. There are often five, ten or even more additives in a single food product. This food, in turn, is often combined with several other additives, to make a single dish.

The casual consumer usually has neither the training nor the interest that would prompt him to attempt an interpretation of the numerous ingredients listed on the label of the average food package. He buys a jar of olives and expects olives; he buys a pound of cold cuts and it never occurs to him to ask about the casing in which the meat is wrapped, nor about the stuff that's injected into them. He's thinking of salad and cold cuts, not a course in chemical preservatives.

For example, let us take the hormone synthetically produced and called for short—stilbestrol. It is widely used in the poultry industry. It is akin to a female hormone. Evidence given to the Delaney Committee in the U.S.A. showed that the danger of producing sterility in humans was far from being the only one. Dr. Robert K. Enders, Professor of Zoology at Swarthmore College stated that it had been conceded that enough of the drug can depress the growth of children, cause cystic ovaries, cystic breasts, cystic kidneys, and suppress ovulation. The "experts" have admitted that minute doses, repeatedly given, are more potentially dangerous than single large doses because of the tendency of drugs to be excreted when given in large doses and accumulated when given in small doses.

"Medical News", November 24,1967, carried a headline which proves our point: "New chemicals kill hundreds". The report continued: "New chemical products were responsible for hundreds of deaths and major epidemics all over the world, an authority on liver diseases warned recently. Scientists admitted, he said, that there were no foolproof tests that they could use to find out if hundreds of new substances used each year would prove poisonous, produce cancers, or result in major genetic damage."

Professor Schmid, Professor of Medicine at the University of California, issued the warning and declared: "We have all these new food additives, preservatives, artificial colorings and taste preservatives. Most of these are non-toxic, but you never know what can happen. We can give rats 100 times the amount humans take in tests that last up to six months, and nothing will happen to the rats. But that does not mean that a tiny amount of the compound taken over twenty years will not produce a cancered man."

What the Hygienists said a long time ago is now being accepted by the establishment—so it seems—from what we read in the London Daily Express of September 10, 1969. It says: "Ten years ago you were a crank if you said that the English ate too much white sugar, starch, and stodge for their health. This week a scientist told the British Association that we are a sluggish, laggard nation, due partly to excessive consumption of high calorie food. Ten years ago you were a crank if you said that excessive use of pesticides was a menace to all forms of life.

Today several pesticides have been banned; and more have been discredited as ultimately ineffectual. And what are today's cranks saying? They're saying that we may be poisoning ourselves with chemical coloring and flavoring in our foods of which we do not yet know the long term effects on human health. And they're saying that if we all had an elementary knowledge of a healthy diet, this nation wouldn't need to spend millions of pounds on drugs every year." Shades of Mohammed walking to the Mountain!— but when will he reach the summit of Hygienic understanding? Will men never learn?

In many ways addition of drugs and chemicals to our food is worse than that of takiing medicines from the chemist. With the latter we can refuse to step into the chemist shop and take his chemical brew; with food additives, the whole community is risking its health and life as with fluoridation of public water supplies.

Because the medical profession, the biologists, and the chemists—so wrapped up around their test tubes and "Bunsen burners"—refuse to recognize the blatant fact that only those substances *that can be utilized by the living body and adapted to its normal metabolic needs are useful to the living organism* and that all other substances that find their way into the organism, by whatever channel, the digestive tract, the lungs, the skin, are not only non-usable, but are positively harmful and toxic, that they are reduced to the necessity of testing each chemical substance individually. If this general fact were accepted by all and sundry, much time, labor and expense involved in this kind of futile research, could be saved. Of greater importance, however, would be the enormous reduction of both animal and human suffering. A blind faith in such a technology must end in self-destruction. Our success has been in building up a technological age, our failure is in the using.

Most people are unwilling victims of the illusion of the invincibility of technology. Their optimism is based on ignorance. The motor car was made before anyone knew about smog, and it is the same with fertilizers and eutrophication, pesticides and bug immunity, detergents, nuclear reactors and food additives. In the beginning there was ignorance—but we are not ignorant now. The danger is staring in our face. To save ourselves we must save the world. This is one of the purposes of writing this book.

In the following pages we wish to give a list of chemical additives *you* the reader eat on an average day if you are living in America. The position in Britain is not far behind. It is imperative that you study it, and may it choke you on your next morsel and make you determined to eat and live Hygienically. This list is by the National Academy of Sciences, National Research Council, Washington 25, D.C., in their publication 398, "The Use of Chemical Additives in Food Processing", February 1956. (Price $2.00).

A List of Chemical Additives
You Eat on an Average Day

BREAKFAST:

Juice—Benzoic Acid (preservative), dimethyl polysiloxane (anti-foaming agent).

Cereal—Butylated hydroxyanisole (antioxidant), Sodium acetate (buffer), FD & C Red −2 (dye), FD & C Yellow +5 (dye), Aluminum ammonium sulfate (acid).

Meat—(sausage, spiced ham, hash), Ascorbate (antioxidant), Calcium phosphate (anti-caking agent), Sodium or potassium nitrate (color fixative), Sodium chloride (Preservative), guar gum (binder).

Toast or Bread—Sodium diacetate (mold inhibitor), Monoglyceride (emulsifier), Potassium bromate (maturing agent), Aluminum phosphate (improver), Calcium phosphate monobasic (dough conditioner), Chloromine T (flour bleach), Aluminum Potassium sulfate (acid-baking powder ingredient).

Buns or

Coffee Cake—Calcium propionate (mold inhibitor), Diglycerides (emulsifier), Sodium alginate (stabilizer), Potassium bromate (maturing agent), Aluminum phosphate (improver), Butyric acid (butter flavor), Cinnamaldehyde Chloramine T (flour bleach), Aluminum potassium sulfate (acid-in baking powder).

Margarine—Sodium benzoate (preservative), Butylated hydroxyanisole (antioxidant) monoisopropyl citrate (sequestrant) FD & C yellow +3 (coloring), Diacetyl (butter flavoring), Stearyl citrate (metal scavenger), Synthetic vitamin A and D.

Butter—Hydrogen peroxide (bleach), FD & yellow +3 (coloring), Nordihydroguaiaretic acid (antioxidant).

Milk—Hydrogen peroxide (bactericide), Oat gum (antioxidant).

Jelly or

Jam—Sodium benzoate (preservative), Dimethyl polysiloxane (anti-foaming agent), Methyl cellulose (thickening agent), Malic acid (acid), Sodium potassium tartrate (buffer), FD & C green +3 (coloring for mint flavors), FD & C yellow +2 (coloring for mint flavors), FD & C yellow +5 (coloring for imitation strawberry flavor), Gum tragacanth (stabilizer).

LUNCH:

Soup—Butylated hydroxyanisole (antioxidant), Dimethyl polysiloxane (anti-foaming agent), Sodium phosphate dibasic (emulsion for tomato soup) Citric acid (dispersant in soup base).

Crackers—Butylated hydroxyanisole (antioxidant), Aluminum bicarbonate (leavening agent), Sodium bicarbonate (alkali), di-glyceride (emulsifing agent), Methylcellulose (bulking agent in low calorie crackers), Potassium bromate (maturing agent), Chloramine T (flour bleach).

Sandwich—Sodium diacetate (mold inhibitor), monoglyceride (emulsifier), Potassium bromate (maturing agent), Aluminum phosphate (improver), Calcium phosphate monobasic (dough conditioner), Chloromine T (flour bleach), Aluminum Potassium sulfate (acid-baking powder ingredient), Ascorbate (antioxidant), Sodium or potassium nitrate (color fixative), Sodium chloride (preservative), guar gum (binder), Hydrogen peroxide (bleach), FD & C Yellow +3 (coloring), Nordihydroguaiaretic acid (antioxidant).

Candy—Sorbic acid (fungistat), Butylated hydroxyanisole (antioxidant), Mono- and Di-glycerides (emulsifying agents), Polyoxyethylene (20) Sorbitan monolaurate (flavor dispersant), Sodium Alginate (stabilizer), Calcium carbonate (neutralizer), Cinnamaldehyde (cinnamon flavoring), Titanimoxide (white pigment), Mannitol (anti-sticking agent), Petrolatum (candy polish), Propyleneglycol (mold inhibitor), Calcium oxide (alkali), Sodium citrate (buffer), Sodium benzoate (preservative).

Soda—Sorbic Acid (fungistat), Sodium benzoate (preservative), Polyoxyethylene (20) sorbitan, monolaurate (flavor dispersant), Sodium alginate (stabilizer), FD & C blue +1 (brilliant blue coloring), FD & C yellow +5 (coloring), Cinnamaldehyde (cinnamon flavoring), Caffeine (stimulant added to cola drinks), butylated hydroxyanisole (antioxidant).

Ice Cream—Mono- and Di-glycerides (emulsifier), Agaragar (thickening agent), Calcium carbonate (neutralizer), Sodium citrate (buffer), Amylacetate (banana flavoring), Vanilldene Kectone (imitation vanilla flavoring), Hydrogen peroxide (bactericide), Oat gum (antioxidant).

DINNER:

Fruit Cup—Calcium hupochlorite (germacide wash), Sodium chloride (prevent browning), Sodium hydroxide (peeling agent), Calcium hydroxide (firming agent), Sodium metasalicate (peeling solution for peaches), Sorbic acid (fungistat), Sulfur dioxide (preservative), FD & C red +3 (coloring for cherries).

Meat—Alkanate (dye), Methylviolet (marking ink), Asafoetida (onion flavoring), Sodium nitrate (color fixative), Sodium chloride (preservative), Sodium ascorbate (antioxidant), Guar gum (binder), Sodium phosphate (buffer), Magnesium carbonate (drying agent).

Canned Peas—Magnesium carbonate (alkali), Magnesium chloride (color-retention and firming agent), Sodium chloride (preservative).

Fruit Pie—Sodium diacetate (mold inhibitor), Sorbic acid (fungistat), Butylated hydroxyanisole (antioxidant), Sodium sulfite (anti-browning), Mono- and de-glycerides (emulsifier), Aluminum ammonium sulfate (acid), FD & C rcd +3 (cherry coloring), calcium chloride (apple pie mix firming agent), Sodium benzoate (mince meat preservative), Potassium bromate (maturing agent), Chloromine T (flour bleach).

(Pie will also contain additives found in shortening and white flour used in making the crust).

Cottage Cheese—Annatto (vegetable dye), cochineal (dye), Diacetyl (butter flavoring), Sodium hypochlorite (curd washing), Hydrogen peroxide (preservative).

Cheese (Processed)—Calcium propionate (preservative), Calcium citrate (plasticiser), Sodium citrate (emulsifier), Sodium phosphate (texturizer), Sodium alginate (stabilizer), Chloromine T (deodorant), Acetic acid (acid), FD & C yellow +3 (coloring), Aluminum potassium sulfate (firming agent), Hydrogen peroxide (bactericide), Pyroligneous acid (smoke flavor).

Beer—Potassium bi-sulfite (preservative), Dextrim (foam stabilizer), Hydrochloric acid (Adjustment of pH), Calcium sulfate (yeast food), Magnesium sulfate (water corrective), Polymixin B (antibiotic).

For the person on a salt-free diet who thinks he is avoiding salt simply by not adding it to his foods in cooking or at the table, the menu will be a sobering revelation. The sodium and chloride compounds he should avoid are present in almost every food he eats. It would be well for anyone restricted against a specific element commonly employed in foods, to study the list of additives given below and carried on labels to be sure that such an element is not contained.

Even if you are careful in selecting the foods you eat, it is practically impossible to live in our civilization without unknowingly eating some food additives. For those who never read a label and try each new work-saving food product that is offered, the chemical intake must be staggering! The only protection you have is to eat as many fresh foods as possible whose origin you know.

The additives mentioned below do not include nonnutritive sweeteners which are used, as suggested by the National Academy of Sciences booklet in: beverages, canned fruit products, canned vegetables, flavoring extracts, frozen desserts, gelatin, jellies, jams, marmalades, baked goods, salad dressings and frozen fruits.

But remember, they could be added to the list of any or all of these foods' additives. The use of glycerols in each food is also not included, but they can be assumed to be present with any flavoring or coloring, for they act as solvents for these items. Isopropanol is another additive we've omitted, but it is contained as a solvent in foods which require synthetic flavoring agents.

Of course, no day's estimate of the foods one eats would be complete without the inclusion of water. Many persons drink eight or more glasses of it each day, and it is the main ingredient of coffee, tea, soda and many other beverages consumed by humans. Those who can get and drink fresh well and spring water, untampered with by engineers who add one chemical after the other to purify metropolitan water supplies, are indeed fortunate. Just for the record, here is a list of the 47 chemicals which are being used by municipal water systems throughout the country to prepare water for us to drink. While it is not likely that all of them would be contained in a single supply, you can be sure that a number of them are in any treated water you might drink. You can add these to the estimate of the chemicals you get every day.

Activated Carbon
Activated Silica
Alum. Ammonium Sulfate
Aluminum Chloride Soln.
Alum. Potassium Sulfate
Aluminum Sulfate
Alum. Liquid
Ammonia, Anhydrous
Ammonia, Aqua
Ammonium Silicofluoride
Ammonium Sulfate
Bentonite
Bromine
Calcium Carbonate
Calcium Hydroxide
Calcium Hypochlorite
Calcium Oxide
Carbon Dioxide
Chlorinated Coperas
Chlorinated Lime
Chlorine
Chlorine Dioxide
Copper Sulfate
Disodium Phosphate

Dolomitic Hydrated Lime
Dolomitic Lime
Ferric Chloride
Ferric Sulfate
Fluosilicic Acid
Hydrofluoric Acid
Ozone
Sodium Aluminate
Sodium Bicarbonate
Sodium Bisulfite
Sodium Carbonate
Sodium Chloride
Sodium Fluoride
Sod. Hexametaphosphate
Sodium Hydroxide
Sodium Hypochlorite
Sodium Silicate
Sodium Sulfite
Sodium Thiosulfate
Sulfur Dioxide
Sulfuric Acid
Tetra-Sod. Pyrophosphate
Tri-Sodium Phosphate

The same chart gives a list of purposes for which these chemicals are used. They are:

Algae Control	Miscellaneous
Boiler Water Treatment	B.O.D. Removal
Colour Removal	Coagulation
Corrosion and Scale Control	Condition-Dewater Sludge Chlorination
Dechlorination	Flotation
Disinfection	Neutralization-Acid
Fluoridation	Neutralization-Alkali
Iron & Manganese Removal	Oxidation
Softening	pH Control
Taste and Odour Control	Reduction

The sweet smell of success of technological food production is beginning to back-fire; one day it will explode and your balloon, dear reader, will go up with it. Hence drink distilled water.

However, I am glad to note that in 1976 the Cancer Research Campaign in Britain in allocating its annual grants, has made a sum of more than £21,000 available to two scientists who are specially concerned with the relationship between certain kinds of cancer and cell-destroying elements in food additives.

Dr. Brian Challis of the Department of Chemistry at Imperial College, London, has been working on sodium nitrate which is added to many protein foods for preservation. It has been noted that nitrosamines have produced malignant tumours in test animals. Dr. Challis has also found out the interesting fact that taking of fresh fruits and vegetables in the diet seem to inhibit the formation of nitrosamines and can therefore be recommended as part of an anti-cancer diet.

A recent estimate of the number of chemical additives used in the food industry is 20,000, the prime objective in most cases being to increase shelf-life in the shops and promote vested interests.

The noted American Nutritionist, Dr. Clive McCay, stated "Fragmentary research is fascinating work; it is comparatively easy to finance it and it can lead to great achievement in scientific reputation and, above all, it is *safe* (Italics)—it does not cut across the established interests of industry, teaching or advertising. The moment you do research into wholes, you find yourself treading on somebody's toes—and they are utterly ruthless, they will knife you and utterly destroy you!"

Hence let us learn to look and not merely to see; to listen and not merely to hear; to relish and not merely to taste; to give and not merely to touch—these are practical means of preventing the deadening habit of taking things for granted.

CHAPTER XIV

Drugs with Anything and Everything

"Since 1914 mankind has been in one of those recurrent moods in which it is bent on going to hell, and since 1945 we have possessed the means of instant conveyance. In this mood human beings are infuriated by a fellow creature who does strive officiously to keep the human race alive in spite of being told he need not.

What business has one man to stay sane when the fashion is to be mad? The intervention is the more exasperating if the self-appointed savior tries to goad us into facing up to our folly by sticking pins deftly into our tenderest spots." (Writing about Bertrand Russell in the London Sunday Telegraph, February 8, 1970, by Arnold Toynbee).

We like the above quotation. It makes us take another look at ourselves and what supposed motive we have of writing such a book as this one—a sort of exposé 1976 style—on the age-old habit of drug-taking. Put it this way: We are fond of this earth, even though it is not always a paradise, and we are equally fond of all its inhabitants, humans included. Having seen the writing on the wall, we wish to contribute something sane and sensible in this mad world where drugs and drugging have taken over the destiny and dignity of the human race. Just as Rachel Carson could not shut her eyes to it, but did what she needs must do, so do we feel that now is the time to give something constructive to millions who are searching for a "Royal Road to Health," and guide others to see the dilemma of drug-taking in all its notoriety.

How much prejudice is maintained from generation to generation because every man must prove to his neighbor that he thinks as he thinks his neighbor thinks? The answer to this is reflected in the attitude of the average individual of our modern-day society to this age-old problem of health and disease.

To what length mankind has gone to search for an answer outside his own self can very easily be seen if one turns the pages of folklore medicine.

But for the tragic sequel in modern times, some of these "old time remedies" reminds us of the humorous, yet pathetic, situations in the old time slapstick comedy films when Charlie Chaplin, Harold Lloyd, and Buster Keaton reigned supreme.

Some time ago there appeared an article in one of the magazines under the title "Green Medicine—A Growing Science." In it was discussed the growing new interests in old plants on the part of the medical profession, and how drug firms are spending large sums of money and sending out pharmacologists into the wilds to hunt for certain weeds to test for their medicinal qualities. It indicates correctly that this change in attitude toward plant substances represents an about-face for a large segment of what it calls "medical science." But it omits to state that this about-face has come as a result of the disastrous effects (so called "side-effects") following the use of synthetic drugs. Briefly going into the history of herbal medicine (the forerunner of present day drug industry) the article fosters the usual myths about healing virtues of poisonous plants. It is the same superstition whatever garb you put on it. People must realize that substances can be toxic and poisonous, no matter whether they be extracted from animal, vegetable, or mineral matter. There are scores of plants (e.g. foxglove from which digitalis is extracted, cinchona bark from which quinine is extracted, the plant from which castor oil is extracted, and so on ad nauseum) which harbor certain toxic substances, and this very quality of the plant is the alleged curative property used in "medicine."

Mineral oil used for constipation by multitudes of people has now been known to cause cancer. In Palm Beach Post, October 19, 1962, appears an article by a physician (Brandstadt) in which he concedes this point. But the cancer is only an end point in a large series of difficulties that result from taking mineral oil. The same applies to poisonous matter, vaccines, serums, hormones made from the animal matter and injected into your blood stream.

We cannot help but repeat and quote an editorial in the

British Medical Journal, August 18, 1962, which said: "The term "side-effect" is probably one of the most misleading terms introduced into medicine. It suggests something so inocuous and incidental that for all practical purposes it can be ignored. The description of a hypersensitivity which may be fatal as a 'side-effect' has possibly made some doctors careless about prescribing, for example, penicillin for relatively trivial conditions. And talking about iatrogenic disease, we may find comforting words to disguise the fact that *this means disease and death caused by the treatment, usually medicinal, doctors give to their patients.*" (Italics mine).

"The more potent drugs which have displaced the innocent medicines in the treatment of many ailments frequently fail to relieve the symptoms which they are intended to control and too often produce their own." This statement was made by Dr. William Evans, M.D., D.S.C., F.R.C.P., writing in the British Medical Journal, September 15, 1962. It points out the medical use of poisons to "relieve" or to "control" symptoms, as though the symptoms are, per se, evils.

We have said before, and we will say it again and again, that in our present day "civilization" almost everything and anything is contaminated by drugs and chemicals of one kind or other. It is like having "chips with everything." We are happy to find some confirmation of our view from authoritative medical sources. We are going to quote from an article entitled, "Toxicology and the Biomedical Sciences" which appeared in the June, 1965 issue of Science, the official organ of the American Association for the Advancement of Science. The high standing of each of the joint authors of this article assures us the last word on the subject.

They say, "The number and variety of chemicals that affect man has increased at an alarming rate and created a public health problem of major proportions. We are confronted with a profusion of chemicals in the form of industrial and municipal wastes, air and water pollutants, herbicides, pesticides, cosmetics, food additives, as well as drugs administered over extended periods of time, and yet we do not know what these substances do to biological systems. In effect, we are thrust into global experiments for which we are not prepared.

"For some of these hazards, such as automobile exhaust fumes or cigarette smoke, we are unlikely to find more compelling evidence of their deleterious effects. It remains for industrial and government bodies to utilize in the public interest all the information now available, and for the scientific community to continue experimentation on the basic mechanisms of their effects and to find ways of preventing or alternating their hazard.

"There remains, however, a major problem with the vast number of chemical compounds whose possible poisonous effects are not known or cannot be predicted. It is this area which is the subject of our article."

Then the authors go on to confirm the Hygienic position that it is futile to test chemical substances, one by one, when it is known that all of them are toxic. Pinpointing this, they say: "It seems futile to record one by one the biological effects of millions of chemical entities without the development of unifying and simplifying generalizations. It is evident that new means must be sought to accelerate the acquisition of new knowledge on the effects of chemicals on living materials, and to develop a system for the rapid dissemination of such information. In this article we outline some of the problems in toxicology and offer recommendations as to how these problems should be approached."

Although these eminent men fully acknowledge that our modern chemical environment is a mass of toxins, and that new and more dangerous toxic substances are continuously being added to our environment, they, as expected, do not offer any obvious and radical a solution as the discontinuance of air pollution, water pollution, food pollution, and countryside pollution with insecticides. As expected the inference is that the increasing poisoning of our environment will continue and that the so-called researchers are to continue testing the various toxins to determine the effects of each.

A few years have passed since that article was written, but up to now we see no obvious solution in sight by the powers that be. Our air in America and Britain is still polluted by fumes containing lead, sulphur dioxide, and other deadly poisons. The results of a quick dose of tetra-ethyl lead have been demonstrated time and again: insomnia, nightmares, restlessness, fear, anxiety, hysteria, insanity, sometimes death. The results of a slow, continuous absorption over a long period of time have never been investigated. Is the human system unaffected, we ask, when it is known that this substance is absorbed by the brain cells, damaging them?

Mental disturbance is accepted today as being as common as the common cold, and what guarantee have we that fuel combustion fumes are not responsible for at least a part of it? Lung cancer is another serious disease rearing its head, and still nothing or very little is being done to have "smokeless zones" free of contamination by fumes shooting from industrial chimneys and laden with sulphur dioxide.

We have already touched upon the food industry and water pollution as well as the pharmaceuticals but how many of us realize the dangers present in turning out glamour by the cosmetic industry? How many realize that the cosmetic industry is part and parcel of the drug industry? The cosmetic art has relied mainly upon chemistry. Even in ancient days Kohol (black antimony) was used by Cleopatra, together with various dyes and paints. In Roman times, oxide of lead was used by many women to whiten their skin, which led to many deaths from lead poisoning and suffering from lead-palsy.

Physicians all through their history have led people up the garden path to believe that drugs can impart beauty as well as health. This ancient practice in camouflaging still persists today. Drugs can no more impart beauty than they can heal. Both are given under wrong pretenses.

Makeup as we now know it, is the development of the last 50 years. Drugging the face is not different from drugging the interior of the woman. The profits in cosmetics are enormous. No amount of grease paint, powder, and color that may be applied to the face and smeared on the lips, however skilfully and artistically done, can hold the enchantment for a man that is contained in a clean face that possesses a clear, fine skin with natural color.

Cosmetic traditions are usually connected with rites of magic, and cosmetic preparations are made of almost anything—clay, poisonous drugs, kangaroo glands, etc.—many of them highly irritating and even destructive to the skin and to the other parts of the body. Drugs for beauty, astringents to "tighten the skin," creams and hormones to reduce or enlarge the breast, preparations to remove wrinkles and warts, to make eyelashes and eyebrows grow, to cure freckles and pimples, etc., convert the cosmetic table into a miniature drug store. Even lipstick is advertised today to heal cracked lips.

Most of these drug cosmetics are not harmless, by any means—what is their long term effect on the health of the skin and the living organism, we ask?

Cosmetics most likely to produce injury are bleaches containing mercury, hair dyes containing metallic and analine compounds, depilators containing sulphides; "pore deep" cleansers containing phenol, (carbolic acid), and powders containing white lead or bismuth. Without a thought, today's women are drugging their face, hair, hands almost continuously. Because the skin constantly comes in contact with harsh, inorganic materials—minerals, petroleum, paraffin waxes, acids, all of which irritates the skin, it deteriorates. The use of such drugging is reflected in pale, pasty, and colorless skin. Mascara and eyelash dyes containing analine dyes, lead, silver nitrate, paraphenylene-diamene, and many other cosmetic drugs have caused much damage, and even blindness, to the eyes.

Gloria Swanson, now in her 70's, has preserved her freshness and beauty without use of lotions or creams.

Depilatories containing tannic acid and other strong chemicals injure the skin and have been known to cause death. Certain types of deodorants cause considerable irritation. Potassium hydroxide, a corrosive poison contained in cuticle removers, often leads to trouble. Corrosive sublimate, a dangerous chemical, is contained in many balms and freckle lotions.

We hear only of the more dramatic effects of this constant poisoning of the skin, and even these are likely to be suppressed in order "not to cause panic" to the public and thus lower their sales. Astringents and tonics for the face usually contain boric acid, sometimes a minute quantity of carbolic acid, and often result in dryness of the skin and other damage. Astringents usually contain alcohol which occasions a mild irritation, referred to as a "pleasant tingling sensation."

The analine base of hair dyes, the lead-and-salt-and-sulphur hair dyes, the harmful substances in freckle removers and in preparations for removal of superfluous hair, the pyrogallol metallic salts in some types of hair dyes, the silver-salt (mercury) dyes, the mercury contained in freckle removers, the analine sulphides, and thallium-acetate in hair removers, the harmful chemicals put into nail polishes and varnish, and the harm and even deaths that have resulted from the use of these substances have not been generally known to the average woman.

Makeup as a substitute for health is funny beyond words. Camouflaging the external evidences of poor health leads to the neglect of health.

Physicians sometimes warn about the dangers in using too much cosmetics, but only when a fatal or dramatic case has occurred and can no longer be suppressed. They admit to the harm contained in the use of such devices but just as they cry "Wolf" with regard to their so-called side-effects—they continue to condone wholesale the practice of cosmetics, just as they condone the use of drugs— in the mistaken belief that both beauty and health can be bought over a drug store counter. They do nothing to condemn and ban the use of either of the practices, but perpetuate this "remedy mentality" for the sake of lucre.

Not long ago arsenic was regarded as a beautifier because it produced transparency of the complexion, brilliance of the eyes, a shapely contour of form, and softness and smoothness of the skin. But the brilliant eye which came about was not the luster of health, but the watery glitter resulting from kidney disease; the clear and transparent skin was but another sign of disease caused by taking this poison; the softly rounded form was not the result of a well nourished and well developed body, but the result of retention of water in the tissues. It was edema. The same arsenic was used in bygone days by horse traders to dose their nags with the poison to give them a rounded appearance, sparkling eyes, and a glossy coat.

Drugs have also been used to rejuvenate us. Hormones and hormone-containing creams are supposed to make young ones out of old ones. This Aladdin fable is no good when it comes to health and beauty. Drugs and drugging is no "Fountain of Youth." Gullible women and men also, who pursue the "Fountain of Youth" in drug stores and "beauty" parlors should have learned long ago that makeup will neither preserve nor restore youth. Older women cannot make themselves look a day younger by the use of such methods. In Britain there is a famous and well-known woman who lends her name and fame to many products guaranteed to restore youth and vigor, but recently when she appeared on television, her face looked old and wrinkled. Yet how many women would see through such deception practised on them? Very few—as the products of such an industry are constantly finding new markets to sell their wares.

Some years ago on March 25, 1970, the London Daily Express quoted Dr. Donald Louria, president of the New York State Council on drug addiction: "Any teenager who smokes 'pot' more than 10 times runs a 1 in 5 risk of getting hooked on more dangerous drugs."

He went on to say, "Surveys in the United States allow us to assess the direct connection between marijuana and other drugs.

"One survey in particular among students showed conclusively that of those who smoked 'pot' once a month, 22 percent went on LSD and other drugs. Of those who smoked once a week, 49 percent went on to stronger drugs. The worst drug inheritance was among those who smoked 'pot' every day—82 percent.

"The general rise in drug abuse relates to the way our society is going. We are pleasure and drug orientated, and as long as we have such ethics, people will fly from one drug to another." (Italics mine, K.R.S.)

Dr. Louria is highly critical of the use of pills—even aspirin—by parents and the effect it has on their children. He says, "The arguments kids use about parents' abuse of cigarettes and booze is a facile rationalisation. It is more the abuse of pills, to sleep, then to awaken, then to slow pain, that impresses them.

"Pill-using parents breed all-taking children." (Italics mine, K.R.S.)

How many parents will try to remember that last phrase of his—when taking their green, yellow, and red pills to restore the magic of youth and beauty to their much abused frames? This is what it is all about, folks—you become used to drugs for everything and anything. You want to excel in athletics, you take Benezedrine before an event. Or you want to slim—why, find the shortest cut to the next chemist and hang the consequences.

But how many realize that such slimming pills are a

danger to life and health? Slimming pills contain drugs affecting the thyroid gland and the whole metabolism of the body. Many comparatively healthy, fat women have been made into invalids by use of such drugs; some of them have even lost their lives. Drugs that are said to "lessen the desire for food" are as dangerous as those that cripple digestion and metabolism. Women are warned against taking these drugs except under the watchful eye of a physician, a warning that should reveal the true character of such substances. By using drugs to reduce, one always runs the risk of permanent injury to the nervous system.

A British paper, "The Guardian", of January 26, 1964, reports a story of a firm in Brooklyn, New York, indicted for making fraudulent claims about a pill which would reduce weight without any sort of dieting. The pill, "Regimen", has now been taken off the market after sixteen million dollars worth of the stuff had been sold.

You want to live longer—stay younger—then there is a drug for you. The Wall Street Journal of April 4, 1964 carries an article on aging. In it we are told of a "juvenile hormone" that was found and, which they hoped would reap a harvest for the manufacturers. What they were interested in was not the cause of aging and a way to avoid these causes or a way to remove them, but a means of wiping out effects without attending to the causes. In other words, the medical approach to every and any human problem is a drug. They must have a drug. Something which the researchers must be able to sell over the counter or injected by a needle. Research today is geared to money making. If it does not make money for those who spend for research, it is a failure.

Researchers must find a way and means within the orbit and life of the individual. Anything that will interfere with the habits and customs of the people is taboo. They must find a filter-tipped cigarette rather than urge the tobacco user to stop smoking. They must find drugs to be infiltrated into our water supply rather than ban the sale of sugar and confectionary. They must find synthetic equivalents of vitamins to "enrich" the flour from which the white loaf of bread is made rather than ban the sale of such flour.

In respect to the enriched white flour, an article in the Lancet, a medical journal, of March 1970, states that it has been found that iron absorption from eating bread made out of whole grain flour is higher than from the best enriched white bread. They could have learned that over a hundred years ago if they had paid attention to Sylvester Graham, a pioneer of Natural Hygiene, who advocated the use of whole grain flour.

Ex-President Johnson, in his State of the Union message on January 7, 1965, deplored the terrible health situation in America, and pleaded for measures to mitigate it. He commented that 48 million then living would become victims of cancer, 15 million would suffer from heart disease; and this together with strokes, accounts for more than half the deaths in the United States each year. 12 million people have arthritis and rheumatic disease and 10 million are burdened with neurological disorders, 5½ million Americans suffer from mental retardation and the number is increased by 126,000 new cases each year; one in five children under age 17 is afflicted with a chronic ailment, 4 million children are emotionally disturbed, four out of five persons 65 or older have a disability or chronic disease, mental illness afflicts one out of ten Americans, fills nearly one half of all the hospital beds in the nation, and costs one billion dollars annually.

What a horrible state of affairs for a country that boasts it has the biggest and best of everything, including medical facilities, physicians, hospitals, gadgets, the lot. Is this what we have to expect from the foremost super-power country in the world? Is this what lies in store for us in Britain and in Europe and Asia? Is this what modern medical science can give us after all the millions spent for research? The answer would be an equivocal Yes—if we let the drug industry and the chemical cartels and the physicians dictate to us.

At the beginning of this chapter we joked about having "chips with everything" but even the chips are back-firing on us now, thanks to the drug industry.

A quarter page advertisement by Universal Oil Products Co. in the Wall Street Journal of January 19, 1966, was a shocking and flagrant reminder of our poisoned food industry. A youngster is shown seated in front of a large bowl of potato chips and underneath is a caption, "Fried nine weeks ago but he will never know." The company boasts that thanks to their discovery of butylated hydroxyanisole, the potato chips taste every bit as good as the day they were made. This is the ingredient, they say, that helps keep many other fat containing foods fresh and free from rancidity.

In simple language, here is an admission that the food is so embalmed with chemicals that no changes can possibly take place in the ingredients.

We have said before that the medical profession is addicted to the absurd idea that instead of finding and removing the cause, the solution is in finding a drug or a chemical. We gave some examples before but here is a beauty, which conclusively proves that this is not just a figment of our imagination but an established fact.

In the Journal of the American Medical Association, June 3, 1961, we read an article which discusses the relation of diet to heart disease and states that recent findings strongly indicate that "a vegetarian diet can prevent 90% of our thromboembolic diseases and 97% of our coronary occlusions." The article stresses the fact that no evidence points to stress as a cause of heart disease, but mentions saturated fat, cholesterol and alcohol, ice cream, butter, eggs, and similar substances as the causes of heart-arterial disease.

Then comes the statement that so graphically confirms our contention. The article says: "Diet is certainly the main factor in achieving protection or in predisposing to early disability and death in clots in veins and clots in plaques in arteries.

"Those who are habituated to diets rich in butter, eggs, and stall-fed pork and beef *know that a doctor's job is to find a drug which will prevent trouble even on the richest diet.* But until a safe way is found to change the metabolism of those prone to vascular disease so that they can handle rich diets in the same way as people with no such weakness, *doctors and even the food industry will have to consider the dietary control of vascular disease as a matter of primary importance.*" (Italics mine, K.R.S.)

Those of you who are new to Natural Hygiene would consider that the intensity of the feelings of those (like the author) who write such books about health and disease, is neurotic. Personally it has never been denied that this may be so. Most of us, nay all of us, grew up in a sick society, and a sick society makes neurotics of one kind and another.

Natural Hygienists the world over can justify this intensity as a need to fling a dramatic challenge to a community they think is moving too slowly, to a society they think is too satisfied with its sins; to fling it like a prophecy; impracticable perhaps, but hopeful of a new world that could come.

One can only face in others what one can face in oneself. On this confrontation depends the measure of our wisdom and compassion. This intense energy is all that one finds in the rubble of vanished civilizations, and to take a personal opinion, it is the only hope of ours.

A few more examples of the follies commited and blunders admitted would see reason prevail. Dr. G. W. Northup, writing in the Osteopathic News of Nov./Dec. 1969, says: "Take the example of a 70 year old patient in a large metropolitan hospital. The internist and other specialists agreed that it was a terminal case. Much to their dismay—so did the patient, who demanded that all medication be discontinued and the various therapies terminated. One of the physicians proclaimed that the patient was voluntarily commiting suicide. But over the protests of the consulting physicians, the patient's will prevailed. The treatment was stopped, and the patient immediately began improving! Admittedly this is an unusual case, but it does drive home the point that overtreatment can often be damaging to the patient."

Another tidbit like the above appears in the medical journal, Lancet, January 3, 1970, where a physician writes and asks: "Is it certain, for instance, that the use of specific drugs for the treatment of pneumonia in the elderly does actually prolong life? Some years ago I had charge of a ward for elderly men in a mental hospital, and I followed a policy of making patients as *comfortable* as possible, without regard for their survival time. Although I have no figures to validate it, I was surprised to get the impression that my patients tended to live longer as a result of this than they would have if I had focused attention upon treating their illnesses." He went on to say: "Professor Mc-Keown has said that the striking increase in life expectation in Britain, which has often been attributed to advances in medical research, has in fact, been mainly a by-product of general social betterment."

Considering the genuine panic among those who are really aware of this drug remedy mentality of every human

situation, we feel the purpose of writing this book is fulfilled, and we are only sorry we did not do the job earlier.
The genuine panic is, of course, that a time is approaching
when "adverse reactions" to drugs will be worse than the
various forms of disease for which they are employed. A
few excerpts taken from the Bulletin of the Atomic Scientists, January 1969, show how seriously is this problem felt
in the U.S.A.

The article with the heading "Drug testing: Is Time
Running Out?" says: "In a survey of 1,014 medical admissions at Yale University's teaching hospital, 10.3 percent
of patients had a drug reaction; in 1.4 percent the reaction
threatened the patient's life; and in 0.4 percent the patient
died as a result of the reaction. A similar survey at Johns
Hopkins of 714 medical patients revealed 17.1 percent had
reactions and 1.55 percent were fatal. Even if only one-
tenth of one percent of all admissions died of drug reactions, the deaths would approach 29,000 per year. Deaths
due to drugs would be a major public health problem comparable in importance to the infectious disease, cancer of
the breast, and nephritis as a cause of mortality."

The London Sunday Telegraph of February 1, 1970, had
also something to say in this respect and equally telling. It
reported that "the American medical-industrial complex
is riding high these days—some would say dangerously
high. Last year $26,250 million went into its collective
pocket—roughly 2½ times what was spent on the Vietnam
War . . ."

However, the sequel to it let the cat out of the bag and
revealed what was obvious to any intelligent person not
beguiled by medical propaganda. It continued: "Boom
days, and with them one would expect a healthier nation
and vast improvements in the standard of care. Yet the
facts are that Americans are not particularly healthy (the
United States ranks 18th in the international life-expec-
tancy charts and 13th in infant mortality), and the patients
are probably the most dissatisfied in the Western world."

The same physician who wrote the article gave instances
of the dangers of some medicines: "I am a specialist in
rheumatic diseases, and through my career I have watched
the development of a series of new drugs for the treatment
of rheumatoid arthritis. I, and many other rheumatologists,
have considerable doubt that any drug is really effective in

arresting the course of rheumatoid arthritis, so surely our first concern should be *prinum non nocre:* first, not to injure the patient. Often it seems, however, that for the long-suffering arthritic the purported cure is worse than the disease.

The article then told us that the patient has very little protection since the doctor often uses very little judgment about the matter. It went on to tell us about the wives of physicians in the United States who gave birth to Thalidomide babies as a result of taking the free samples sent to their husbands, and the point was stressed that doctors may be wary about notifying drug reactions since to do so might involve them in legal disputes. "We do not know the extent to which adverse reactions to drugs are a problem in American society, and probably we will never know since the physician and the drug company both attempt to conceal evidence of toxicity."

The concluding remark was: "All the elements for vast future catastrophies are present: lots of new, highly toxic drugs, sloppy and dishonest testing, and hard-sell, dishonest advertising campaigns, to which the average physician is highly susceptible."

If such a charge had been made by a Hygienist, he would have been hounded out of the country by an all powerful medical lobby—one wonders what penace was demanded from this medical man who expressed his opinion in public.

In a book published in 1975 by a Penguin special called "There's Gold in them thar Pills—An inquiery into the medical Industrial complex" (Author Alan A. Klass BA. M.D. FRCS) We find the following exerpt which sets the tone of the theme presented.

"Who else but the individual doctor true to his Hippocratic oath, can support the ill in their unequal contest with an agressive profit motivated, multinational industry? If enough are willing, they may be a powerful enough force to change the course of the multinationals. This is something that the medical association had no wish to do and Governments have failed to do. Individual doctors have only to say no loudly and clearly."

The book is a fascinating story by Dr. Klass of how the drug industry has spread its influence over the profession: how drug advertising sustains the life of medical journals and how further education of physicians, nurses and medical auxilliaries is done by Seminars, Conferences, meetings and printed matter all arranged by the drug companies.

In our virus and germs bogey society, a reading of a book "Life on Man" by Theodore Rosebury can be enlightening to those who would be prepared to read between the lines. You have a cut finger, a bleeding wound from a stray bullet, or grazed your knee while playing football. Then you just have to wait a few minutes to apply some iodine, Dettol, mercurochrome, or some such other drugs, and you have licked the viruses and germs.

But Dr. Rosebury points out with great emphasis, that if bacteria which abide in such huge numbers in the body were enemies, no human being would have lived to draw a few breaths. So the author rightly asks, why do we feel compelled to do silly things like slip a bag marked "sanitized" over a drinking glass, or invest money and time in mouthwashes, iodine and other antiseptics?

Dr. Rosebury agrees with the Hygienic approach when he says that iodine strong enough to clean the germs out of a wound would damage tissue and kill the scavenging cells that were mobilized to sop up the microbes anyway. Bacteria seem to belong in and on man, is Dr. Rosebury's view. We commence to accumulate them immediately after birth, he states, and in exchange for living off us in uncountable numbers, they render us services. Rosebury points out that animals brought up in a germ-free environment are miserable creatures with enfeebled hearts and sluggish undeveloped intestinal tracts.

So more than a century later we have arrived at a full circle where the words of the eminent French physician and physiologist, Professor Majendie, ring true. This is what he said in one of his lectures to medical students in the middle of the last century: "Gentlemen, medicine is a great humbug . . . Doctors are merely empirics when they are not charlatans."

And Sir John Forbes, F.R.C.S., who was then physician to the Queen's Household, wrote in the British and Foreign Medical Review in 1846: "In a large proportion of cases treated by allopathic physicians, the disease is cured by nature and not by them. For less, but not a small proportion, the disease is cured by nature in spite of them. In other words, their interference opposes instead of assists the case. Consequently, in a considerable proportion of diseases, it would fare as well or better with patients, in the actual condition of the medical art as now generally practiced, if all remedies, at least active remedies, especially drugs, were abandoned."

What was written a hundred or more years ago is not just ancient history, but still true today in the field of drug taking. Since then, no valid scientific foundation for the administration of drugs has been discovered. We see more and more serious "side-effects" from the new than from the older drugs; we see a greater number of deaths from "allergy" to drugs than in the past; we see a greater army of chronic sufferers, with an ever increasing incidence of degenerative diseases; we see less and less attention to prevention of disease and health building, and more and more attention devoted to patching up symptoms till another day. In 1935 a French physician and physiologist, a Nobel prize winner, wrote his famous book, "Man the Unknown" and confessed for the medical profession of the entire world, the inadequacies of the art of drugging. Where then lies this evidence of progress?

The following words of Dr. Carrel are as true today in 1976 as it was in 1935. Let us read them all over again: "Medicine is far from having decreased human suffering as much as it endeavors to make us believe. Indeed, the number of deaths from infectious diseases has greatly diminished, but we still must die, and we die in a much larger proportion from degenerative diseases. The years of life which we have gained by the suppression of diphtheria, smallpox, typhoid fever, etc., are paid for by the long suffering of the lingering deaths caused by chronic infections, and especially by cancer, diabetes, and heart disease."

Can we, the Natural Hygienists, be blamed for opening our mouths and shouting from the roof tops? We should be thankful, too, that we live in an age of mass communication when a small group with something definite and positive to say has a chance of reaching a wider audience with their message via this book and other such Hygienic publications.

Earlier civilizations could decline in relative peace and leave their faults uncorrected until they became uncorrectable. The voices of protest were not heard above the din of revelry, and if they grew too strong they could always be silenced.

Our generation now enjoys the benefit of feedback—the scientist term for the governor that regulates the modern technical process of production. This book and other Hygienic publications are our feedback system, telling us that something is wrong when there is still time to put it right.

Can we sit tight with compressed lips and folded hands when we see such items as "It is a ludicrous paradox that millions of women are swallowing daily a drug known to produce effects which doctors spend much of their time trying to prevent in other patients," from the Observer March 1, 1970, as uttered by Professor Victor Wynn, in relation to the contraceptive pill.

Or "The habit of prescribing aspirin for febrile illnesses is deeply rooted in the medical profession, but have we asked ourselves whether this is logical and whether it may be harmful? As I see it, the rise in temperature in a febrile illness is a defense mechanism against the bacterium or virus—Might not some of the prolonged illness after influenza be due to the habit of trying to 'sweat it out' with antipyretics?", from a doctor writing in the British Medical Journal of January 3, 1970.

Is his not an indictment against those who peddle drugs for our health's sake?

Modern advertisers by cunning and subtle methods have been the "hidden persuaders" in getting the people to buy useless and worthless things, lulling them with a false sense of security. When an individual or a nation is drained of its energy, is it a wonder that both the human and material resources of a country are steadily declining?

Most manifestos are ephemeral things—the products of some passing crisis, they quickly lose their interest and lie yellowing in a public library awaiting the attention of a distant historian. But Natural Hygienists believe that their manifesto has more permanent value. It has arisen from the hearts and consciences of men and women who have brooded long and silently over the development of events and who finally can hold their peace no longer. When they speak, they speak with the force and power that comes from accumulated experience and deeply held convictions.

Instead of flogging their skills and imaginations to sell such things as artificial sweeteners, stomach powders, hair restorers, fluoride-toothpaste, before-and-after shave lotions, slimming pills, tonics, deodorants, fizzy water, filtered cigarettes, roll-ons, pull-ons, slip-ons, chocolate laxatives, sugared quinines, black-currant pastilles, hi-protein concentrates, vitamins, aspirins, Beechams powders, Alka-Seltzers, Bell-tums, starch-free rolls, and many other far too numerous to mention, they devote their time, space, and energy in selling, nay, giving their knowledge and experience of health laws. The time and effort of those working in the advertisement industry is wasted on those trivial purposes, which contribute little or nothing to the prosperity of any nation.

In common with an increasing number of the general public, the Natural Hygienists have reached the saturation point at which the high pitched scream of consumer swelling is no more than sheer noise. They think that there are other things more worth using their skill and experience on. Since this is a world full of advertisement, they are out to sell and promote to their fellow human beings a greater awareness of the world they live in. They are proposing a reversal of priorities in favor of the more useful and more lasting, instead of those of the synthetic environment of the twentieth century. They hope that their society will tire of gimmick merchants, status persuaders and the like, and put first things first. They are the avant-garde holding the warning light—they may be passed over but they will have the satisfaction of not having the accusing finger of promoting false values pointed at them.

The measure of a man is what he did and does to others. Must the clear stream of their charity be fouled by the scum of taunts and insults from those who have done less? The essence of Natural Hygiene is that knowledge and healing is within us and that we reach both by peeling off the various illusions as one does an orange.

Yes, Sir, getting at the truth is a high class form of strip tease, and Natural Hygienists recommend that it should be a daily practice for all in front of a self-revealing mirror—then as the poet Tagore says: "When one knows thee, then alien there is none, then no door is shut."

CHAPTER XV

Drugs and Cancer

". . . How far should we go, or try to go, in compounding drugs for our society? This suggests an allied and somewhat broader question: Are we indeed trying to work with Nature, or are we trying to work against and control it?

"In the world at large, with all the vast technologies and powers now available, it would appear that man is moving along rather complacently in the belief that he will one day conquer Nature and bring all its forces under his control. Perhaps he will. On the other hand, there is evidence that he is not controlling Nature at all, but distorting it . . . his powers have extended so far that Nature itself, formerly largely protective, at least in the long historical or biological view, seems to have become largely retaliatory. Let man make the smallest blunder in his far-reaching and complex physical or physiological reconnections, and nature, striking from some unforeseen direction, exacts a massive retribution." (Dickinson W. Richards, Nobel Laureate in Medicine, 1956, in "Drugs in our Society", edited by Paul Thalaley and published in 1964).

As long ago as 1775 a London physician by the name of Percival Pott observed that chimney sweeps got scrotal cancer and linked it with their occupation. Chemical carcinogenesis thus came into the picture.

One hundred and forty years later in 1915 two Japanese research workers, Jamagiva and Itshikawa, demonstrated that tumors can be experimentally induced with coal tar in animals. Since then it has been known that a wide variety of chemical agents can cause cancer in both laboratory animals and man.

The late Sir Earnest Kennaway and his colleagues at the Royal Cancer Hospital were the first to prepare carcinogenic compounds in pure chemical form. These were aromatic polycyclic hydrocarbons of the type thought to be responsible for the carcinogenicity of coal tar and of various mineral oils. From 1935 and then onwards many different types of chemical carcinogens have come to light. These include the aromatic amines and aminostilbenes, urethene, many different biological alkylating agents, various metals, such as nickel, iron, beryllium, chromium and arsenic, and minerals such as asbestos and numerous azo dyes. Recently several new classes of carcinogens have been discovered, such as a whole range of different nitrosanimes and lactones.

In our present day and age, man encounters potentially carcinogenic chemical agents in every part of his environment. In previous chapters we have shown that agricultural chemicals such as herbicides, insecticides, and fertilizers contaminate our food. Also that numerous chemicals such as emulsifiers, anti-oxidants, stabilizers, and colors are added to food for so called "preservation" or product appeal.

During the roasting or frying of food, a carcinogen, 3-4 benzpyrene, is formed. The same chemical is present in smoked food. Hence the Hygienist condemns such methods of cooking and prefers to eat his food as much as possible in the raw state. If any cooking is to be done, it should be done with the minimum of time and great heat and conservatively cooked.

At home, man inhales numerous dusts and sprays in the course of household maintenance, or in toilet preparations and cosmetics. Some of the drugs and pharmaceutical preparations in his medicine chest and prescribed by a regular qualified physician are potentially carcinogenic. The creosote with which he preserves his garden fences is strongly carcinogenic for mice.

In his occupation, be he miner, painter, motor mechanic, etc., man is exposed to certain chemical agents which have demonstrated very dramatically that cancer can be an occupational hazard.

Let us classify potential cancer hazards from food.

"(1) Constituents of natural foods (for example: Major constituents, such as cycasin and bracken; minor constituents such as safrote and citrus oils; breakdown products due to ripening or general decay; carcinogenic constituents produced by contamination with specific microbes and the production of toxins by them, such as aflatoxin; toxin produced by penicillin is landicum).

(2) Carcinogens introduced during cooking (for example, carcinogens produced by the overheating of fats; 3-4 benzpyrene in smoked foods, coffee and charcoal steaks).

(3) Contamination of foods with man-made chemicals (for example: insecticides, such as D.D.T., aldrin, dieldrin and aramite; herbicides, fertilizers, hormones, such as estrogens; antibiotics, detergents, metals, such as tin, lead, selenium, etc.).

(4) Chemicals used in food preservation and processing (for example: stabilizers, anti-oxidants, anti-foaming agents; emulsifiers, dispersing agents, preservatives).

(5) Substances added deliberately to food for purpose of flavor or color (for example: sweeteners such as dulcin, saccharin, and cyclamates, numerous other flavors, colors such as butter yellow, poncean 3 Rand blue VRS).

(6) Carcinogens introduced into food as a result of sterilization by ionizing radiation."

These facts were culled from a book, "The Prevention of Cancer" by Drs. R. W. Raven and F. J. C. Roe. The same writers, however, go on to say that "Any proposal to expand the testing of food constituents for carcinogenicity should be viewed in perspective, as even the strictest legislation cannot hope to exclude all carcinogens from food." From this it is quite obvious that the medical profession is aware of the dangers of causation of cancer from drugtaking, but are unwilling to ban all drugs and prefer to take risks.

However, Dr. R. A. Holman, M.D., senior lecturer in Bacteriology, School of Medicine, University of Wales, and Honorary Consultant Bacteriologist to the United Cardiff Hospitals, comes nearer to the Hygienist viewpoint in an article published in the Soil Association Magazine "Mother Earth" and which was based on the paper he read to the International Conference on Nutrition and Vital Substances in September 1961. This is what he says: "It is now almost 50 years since experiments were done which demonstrated that certain chemical compounds could produce tumors in experimental animals, and since that time the emphasis has been on the attempt to determine those agents which are the most carcinogenic (cancer-causing).

But it is now accepted by well informed opinion that almost any form of long continued maltreatment of the cell may result in the development of cancer. The only sensible way to look at cancer from the point of view of causation is to consider the common denominator for all the agents—and that is the cell upon which they act.

"Normal cells can be made to go malignant when exposed to a wide range of unrelated physical and chemical agents. One of the few well-established facts about cancer is that the important enzyme, catalase, is progressively diminished in the host as well as in the tumor. Catalase inhibition is known to be associated with mutagenic processes and the development of viruses, and it is known that many of the proven carcinogenic agents can inhibit this enzyme. In fact, catalase inhibition in red blood cells has been suggested as a rapid method of screening agents for carcinogenic activity.

"It is now realized that the widespread distribution of catalase in living cells is essential for their ability to live aerobically. Just as with bacteria, it is very probable that there is a specific catalase-peroxide balance for each type of animal cell, and if this is interfered with for a sufficiently long time, then abnormal biochemistry occurs which could lead to the development of cancerous cells."

He then goes on to say: "Since many physical and chemical agents can alter the catalase-peroxide balance, and some of these are cumulative, then the prevention of cancer, which must be our ultimate goal, can be realized if we see to it that our cells have a high concentration of catalase and that this is not depleted over the years by exogenous and endogenous factors. Dr. Berglas (author of 'Cancer—Nature, Cause and Cure'—L'Institute Pasteur, Paris), regards as Utopian that we can reverse trends of civilization in this respect, a truly defeatist attitude. But I believe, just as others like the Nobel Prize winners, Alexis Carrel and Szent-Gyorgi, have pointed out in the past, that until we intelligently reform some of our habits of civilization, there will be no measurable reduction in the incidence of this disease.

"The plan of attack for the prevention of cancer should be threefold: (1) to increase our intake of catalase, (2) to increase the manufacture of catalase by our own cells, and (3) to curtail the intake of agents which destroy or inhibit our cell catalase.

(1) To increase our intake of catalase. Civilized man now lives primarily out of the can, the bottle, and the package. Most of the foodstuffs in these are practically sterile. The fear of the microbe has gone too far, and it is now high time that, whilst being on guard for certain pathogens, we should view the majority of organisms in a different light. The agents used to destroy the bacteria invariably destroy or inhibit the catalase in the food. Man is the only species of animal now deliberately taking a large part of his food in a form devoid of catalase. It would be to everyone's great advantage if the consumption of fresh fruits and vegetables were to be markedly increased, thus ensuring an adequate intake of catalase and peroxidase.

(2) To increase the manufacture of catalase by our own cells. It was shown many years ago that, if a normally active creature is forcibly imprisoned in a cage so as to limit its normal muscular activity, then after some weeks the catalase content of the body decreases. Conversely, normally inactive creatures can be made to develop more catalase if forcibly exercised. It is my contention that the chronic habit of limiting the muscular activity of man by encouraging him to imprison himself in cars, trains, and other forms of mechanical locomotion, is doing much to diminish his normal catalase level. This one habit, coupled with the widespread, unphysiological practice of relying upon external heat in the form of electric blankets, central heating, etc., is doing a great deal of damage in decreasing the ability of our cells to respond to those normal stimuli which reflexly induce the synthesis of catalase. Priig has already shown that, according to our daily habits, the body catalase level varies, and it is therefore of the utmost importance that our normal animal physiology must be considered when designing our civilized way of living. In general, a higher concentration of catalase implies an increased consumption of oxygen, which provides a catalytic system of prime importance in the detoxication of our bodies."

From a Hygienic standpoint the pathology of cancer is an evolving one and a sort of end result to the gross misuse of the living organism. Toxemia, the basic cause of disease, has so evolved as to reach an end point so that a state of irreversible condition is soon reached. Anything which builds up toxemia by enervating habits, hastens the evolution of such a pathology.

Many drugs, chemicals, etc. put a great deal of strain on the liver, and the liver being a great detoxifying organ when it breaks down is unable to do its job efficiently and helps then to the evolution of toxemia. Dr. Kasper Blond, another enlightened medical physician, believed that the breakdown of the liver was in many cases the beginning of cancer pathology. He put forth his ideas in two books, "The Liver and Cancer—a New Cancer Theory" (1955) and "Liver Damage as the Cause of Cancer and all Pre-cancerous Conditions" (1960).

Appropriate to the above, it is interesting to read in The Lancet, May 19, 1962, that: "The liver is the first organ which a drug reaches after its absorption from the gastro-intestinal tract, and it is also the main site of the mechanisms of detoxication. It is therefore not surprising that reports are accumulating of toxic liver injury associated with a bewildering variety of new and highly potent drugs."

That cancer is a disease of civilization has now been accepted by most, other than some die-hard stubborn people. A report published in Osteopathic News, September 15, 1963, reveals that there are people living in some parts of the world who are not afflicted with cancer. Investigating some Indians who live in Mexico and who subsist mainly on the corn they grow, the report says: "There has been no recorded case of cancer or any other malignancy among the Tarahumara Indians over the past 40 years, during which time medical records have been kept. Perhaps it is the altitude they live at, the soil they grow their corn in, or their diet. Perhaps it is a combination of three factors."

Sir Robert McCarrison, the famous nutritionist, found a similar situation when in the early years of his life he was a physician in the Hunza Valley (now part of Pakistan) bordering on Kashmir and the Himalayas.

Let us therefore quote some more of what Dr. Hohnen, M.D., has to say because we believe that he is on the right track, in relation to his ideas on cancer prevention. He continues: "(3) to curtail the intake of agents which destroy or inhibit our cell catalase. This is probably the most important mode of attack. In a recent paper the writer described the main exogenous factors to which man is now being deliberately exposed as a result of his very artificial environment. As others have pointed out, civilization is becoming toxic in every sense of the word, and as man reproduces his species relatively slowly, it will take many thousands of years for him to adapt, if this is ever possible.

The toxic agents can be summarized briefly according to the mode of entry into the body, Viz. ingestion, inhalation, injection, or irradiation.

Ingestion. During the past 50 years many diverse alien chemicals have been added to food and drink. It has been estimated that there are now more than 1,000 such agents. Many of these interfere with the catalase-peroxide balance, e.g. sulphur dioxide, sodium nitrate, sodium fluoride, certain hormones, insecticides, fungicides, and dyes.

"In the writer's opinion, most of the chemicals added to food and drink for preservation or coloring could and should be abolished. The obvious way to preserve food is to make use of energy provided by atomic power for deep-freeze transportation and storage. This would ensure a non-toxic food supply with many vital enzyme systems intact (assuming, of course, that the foodstuffs are not covered or impregnated with toxic chemicals as a result of spraying, etc.).

The deliberate addition of the rat-killer, sodium fluoride, to public water supplies with the intent of delaying the onset of dental caries is a most unscientific and unethical measure. Sodium fluoride is a potent catalase poison and is cumulative. The use of sodium fluoride is fraught with danger, and in any case it does not deal with the prime cause of dental caries, which is generally recognised as being a sophisticated and chemically adulterated food supply.

The indiscriminate consumption of catalase-destroying drugs by the civilized races is a matter of serious import. Antipyretics, sulphanomides, barbiturates, and certain tranquilizers are all known to interfere with the catalase-peroxide mechanism.

Inhalation. The majority of the poisonous chemicals which pollute the oxygen that is so vital for our health have been placed there by man. Vast amounts of sulphur dioxide and sulphuretted hydrogen—two very potent catalase poisons—are released daily into our environment as a result of burning fuels of various kinds. Many other toxic chemicals are ejected into the effluents from furnaces, fires, railroad and sea transports, as well as from tobacco smoking. Some of these fumes contain agents which interfere with catalase; e.g. 3-4 benzpyrene.

"The indiscriminate use of aerosols containing insecticides, fungicides, antibiotics, etc., on farms and in domestic institutions is a matter of deep concern to us all. Many of these agents interfere with the respiration of cells via the catalase-peroxide mechanism. Their use on such a wide scale is fraught with danger.

It is obvious that the control of air pollution demands our most urgent attention.

Injection. Modern therapy of disease processes relies to a large extent on the injection of drugs. The sulphanomides, which have been known for a long time to inhibit catalase in vivo and two of which are proven carcinogens, have been widely used for almost 30 years. Who can tell what part these have played in increasing the incidence of leukemia in children or cancer in adults?

Many drugs now used can interfere with cell respiration, and there is an urgent need for work to be done in this field before we can asses the long term risk.

Irradiation. X-Rays and other forms of irradiation are known to inhibit catalase. X-Rays have helped enormously in elucidating certain aspects of disease but, like most other key discoveries in nature, these have been widely applied for decades without the mechanism of action being understood.

At last we now realize that we do not know the threshold below which these rays cease to be harmful, and many authorities are advising the curtailment of mass X-Ray programs as well as the limiting of individual dosage.

There are many other forms of man-made radiation which are being placed on, around, and in us. What effect these will play in increasing the cancer incidence 20 years hence is unknown, but we have been warned repeatedly about letting this problem get out of hand.

"In conclusion, it can be said that the greatest problem in medicine which faces man today is the disease which we call cancer. *This is the result of chronic interference with the fundamental catalase-peroxide mechanism of our own cells brought about by our own folly.* The answer to this disease is to have all energies focused on the preventive aspect. To this end, it is urgently required that a concentrated effort be made at international level to curtail the intake of catalase-inhibiting agents, *whether in the air, food, drink, drugs, or radiation to which we are exposed.* This plan should be coupled with a *campaign to increase the intake of catalase by the consumption of fresh, living foodstuffs, together with a re-education of man to use his animal body in the way for which it was designed.*

Cancer prevention can show results—*if we pull together and reform some of the bad habits so prevalent in our civilized way of living.*" (Italics mine, K.R.S.)

The Hygienists have been saying more or less the same thing that Dr. Holman spoke of—for a long number of years. It is heartening to know that there are some honest people about in the medical profession and who are ready to speak out so openly. The Hygienic movement has had such notable people as Dr. Isaac Jennings (1798-1859), Dr. William Alcott, Dr. Russell Thacker Trall, Dr. John H. Tilden, M.D. (1851-1940), Dr. George S. Weger, and others who were qualified physicians of their era and who saw through the art and practice of medicine and embraced the Hygienic cause.

In olden days there used to be something called "The divine right of kings," whereby it was accepted that "the King can do no wrong." It was for this idea that King Charles I of England lost his head, after which "the divine right" fell into the discard of history, and is now almost forgotten.

But there is still a certain section of the community which adopts the self-same attitude of omniscience and omnipotence and who claim for themselves that "they can do no wrong"—namely, the medical profession.

Not that they, as a body, or as individuals, make any such claim; it is merely that they act on the principle in question, and the Governments and public alike fully accept it and all that it implies. The process is unspoken and unconscious, as it were, but nonetheless it is there, as the pages of the press bear testimony every day.

It is therefore cold comfort for us to be told that our bodies have a lower concentration of various injurious drugs and chemicals and that it is safe to take them into our bodies up to a given point. Who draws the line of safety and where do we draw it?

Reading from the Annual Abstract of Statistics in 1966 we find that in England and Wales during the ten years from 1955 to 1965 there has been a steady increase in the incidence of leukemia and aleukemia, malignant neoplasm of the breast, malignant neoplasm of the trachea, bronchus, and lung, and malignant neoplasm of other sites, and that there have been significant increases in congenital malformations (17 percent over the decade), and vascular lesions affecting the central nervous system (11 percent over the 10 years).

It is difficult to believe that such an increase "just happened" for in the same handbook a list of so-called *permitted* additives is provided.

In relation to cosmetics, a soothing note of control creeps in as we read that "In spite of the progress made, some carcinogens are probably still present in toilet or cosmetic preparations. Not all the dyes used in lipstick and other materials have been subjected to adequate biological tests. Chloroform, which induces liver tumors in mice, still appears to be added to some toothpastes as a flavor.

Estrogens are used in some skin creams. The eurotax group approved of the use of these preparations, provided that they were used only by women aged over 30 years, that they did not contain more than 350 international units of estrogenic hormone per gram, and that not more than 15 grams of the preparation were used per week. The administration of even small amounts of estrogen to postmenopausal women might facilitate the growth of hormone-dependent mammary cancer; hormone creams, therefore, should not be used by such subjects.

There is no doubt that the careless use of cosmetics and other toilet preparations could be a contributory cause of cancer, and their use should be controlled, to avoid all health hazards." (From "The Prevention of Cancer" chapter on cosmetics, written by E. Boyland).

The same source, "The Prevention of Cancer", gives us varied information on well known drugs in a common usage which may be potentially carcinogens and dangerous. Sulphanomides, penicillins, chlonamphenicol, streptomycin, actinomycins, ciriseofulvin, isonicotinic acid hydrazide, arsenic, iron, urethane, silver and gold, phenylbutazone, tar and creosote, medicinal paraffin, thiouracil, 131I, cortisone, corticosteroids, estrogens, progestational agents, including contraceptives, tannins, 8-hydroxyquinoline (a constituent of some spermicidal contraceptive preparations and of skin ointments), implanting of foreign materials in the course of plastic surgery e.g. polyvinyl sponge, all are suspect. The most telling paragraph reads: "It is a well known paradox that many of the chemical agents currently used in the treament of cancer are themselves carcinogenic. Virtually all the commonly used alkylating agents, including the simple nitrogen mustards, HN2 and HN3, treatamine (TEM), chlorambucil, sarcolysin and melphalan, and busulphan (myleran) can induce cancer fairly readily in experimental animals."

Also "It would be easy to assume, on the basis of present evidence, that current prescribing habits entail little risk of carcinogenesis. However, one should bear in mind that the new cases of cancer we see today might be attributable to medical treatment given more than 20 years ago, and that the dangers of what we prescribe today may not be manifest for a similar period."

Must we then wait for such a time when it is too late to do anything? Must "the divine right of doctors-physicians" remain unchallenged, carrying with it the acceptance of the idea that "the medical profession can do wrong," despite the all-too-numerous instances—recounted in the press itself—which refute the belief?

The reader should not be misled into thinking, from what has been said, that we would like the public to transfer their belief "in the divine right of doctors" into a corresponding belief in "the divine right of Natural Hygienists"! Far from it; such beliefs are best dropped completely. They spring from a childish faith. What should replace the old belief is the realization that all men are human and fallible, and that the cure of disease is not something which depends upon a certain section of the community having more than human powers, but rather on thte ability to understand what disease is, and how it can be prevented and successful recoveries made from ill health, by applying the fundamental requisites of life.

In the words of Sir William Slater, writing in his book, "Man must Eat" (University of Chicago Press, 1964), what we must remember is that "The danger lies not in the past, where by good fortune nature has protected man from his own folly, but in the future, where the folly might be so great that the protective mechanism would be of no avail."

Those of you who feel that writers of Natural Hygiene are promoters of anxiety and label us as scaremongers, must remember that we have abandoned the criteria set by the medical profession, not out of sheer cussedness but because we have in the first place tried the medical way and found it deploringly wanting. As Thomas Hobbes wrote in 1651: "But this is certain; by how much one man has more experiance of things past than another; by so much also he is more prudent and his expectations the seldomer fail him."

According to the Times, October 7, 1974, there are more than 30,000 operations for Breast Cancer in Britain, and more than 10,000 deaths. At the present time, so far as treatment is concerned, it is argued that the sooner surgery is used the better chance there is of survival, a view contradictory to the findings of Natural Hygiene. That assumes, of course that the disease has already developed beyond the preventative stage. However according to an Editorial in The Lancet a medical journal of September 21, 1974 the drugs are one of the causes of Breast Cancer developing: "Three articles in The Lancet report a suspected association between rauwolfia therapy and breast cancer. Doctors and governments face some difficult decisions. The rauwolfia alkaloids were introduced into Western clinical practice in the mid-1950s for the treatment of psychosis and hypertension. They are derived primarily from the roots of the shrub Rauwolfia serpentina, which is indigenous to India and neighboring countries. In fact, their use in psychosis is described in ancient Hindu writings, whilst the hypertensive action was described in an Indian medical journal in 1931. 'It is interesting to note that the three articles referred to were from the U.S., Finland and the U.K., and they all agreed that the link between the drugs and the disease 'was a distinct possibility'."

The editorial summed up by saying: "What implications do these findings have then for the use of rauwolfia? Do its therapeutic advantages outweigh the reported cancer risk? In many cases the initial answer must be "No", and in the next few weeks most doctors must surely be reviewing their patients on these agents and reflecting on possible alternative treatments—or no treatment."

Unfortunately, this is another example of a remedy being in use for many years before its possible dangers are realised, and it raises the perennial problem of drug therapy: while a drug may be apparently useful in treating one form of disease it may provoke another more disastrous one—as the above report tends to show.

Another report towards the end of November 1974 reported that American Government Officials undertook urgent tests of drinking water throughout the U.S.A. prompted by a medical report which connected the chlorine used in cleaning and disinfecting drinking water with the generation of cancer and other diseases.

Now a report in the paper "Midnight" September 1st, 1975, screams with the headlines "Cancer cures more deadly than Disease". It goes on to say: "Treatment for cancer will kill you a lot sooner than if nothing were done at all, claims a prominent Cancer researcher."

"My Studies have proved conclusively that untreated cancer victims actually live up to four times longer than treated individuals" DR. Hardin B. Jones told MID-NIGHT.

"For a type of cancer, people who refused treatment lived for an average of 12½ years. Those who accepted Surgery and other kinds of treatment lived an average of only three years! "Beyond a shadow of doubt, radical Surgery on Cancer patients does more harm than good." As for radiation treatment—"Most of the time it makes not the slightest difference wether the machine is turned on or not."

Dr. Jones a psysiologist with the University of California Dept. of medical Physics, has been studying Cancer for more than 23 years. He has travelled the world collecting data on the dreaded disease, and presented his findings to the American Cancer society and medical Schools. Asked why the medical world has ignored his findings, he replied: "Frankly, I don't know the reasons. But they probably become caught up in the tidal wave of individuals demanding treatment."

This has been shown especially in the type of bone cancer—osteogenic Sarcoma—that affects the large knee knee joints, DR. Jones said. Senator Edward M. Kennedy's son, Ted Jr., suffered from that disease and his affected leg was amputated.

A Surgeon is tempted to amputate, just for the relief of pain, DR. Jones noted. "But unfortunately it seems to be only a quesion of time, usually, before the disease pops up again all over the body. "I attribute this to the traumatic effect of Surgery on the body's natural defence mechanism," he said.

The body has a natural defence against every type of cancer, DR. Jones maintained.

"Medical treatment seems to interfere with and mess up this natural resistence" he said.

"You see, it is not the cancer that kills the victim. It's the breakdown of the defence mechanism that eventually brings death." DR. Jones said he advocates less Surgery and Chemotheraphy. (Drugs treatment. K.R.S.) And he pooh-poos what he said were claims by the medical profession of certain cancer "cures". The fact remains, said DR. Jones, that just as many people die today from cancer as they did in the year 1900. The mortality rate hasn't changed much. "With every Cancer patient who keeps in excellent physical shape and boosts his health to build up his natural resistance, there's a high chance the body will find its own defence against the cancer," he said.

"He may have many good years left in good health. He shouldn't squander them by being made into a hopeless invalid through radical medical intervention, which has zero chance of extending his life."

DR. Jones agreed that lumps in the breast should be checked out. "But it's utter nonsense to claim that catching cancer symptoms early enough will increase the patient's chances of survival," he said. "Not one medical scientist or study has proven that so in any way".

Furthermore untreated breast cancer cases show a life expectancy four times longer than treated ones, he averred.

"My wife and I have discussed what she would do if breast cancer was diagnosed in her", DR. Jones continued. "And we both agree she would do nothing as regards treatment, except to keep as healthy as possible.

"I guarantee she would live longer! "For not only does radical Surgery or chemotheraphy do nothing to prolong a cancer victim's life, but that same victim will, in most

cases, live a lot longer if he or she refuses treatment."
As if to corroborate what DR. Hardin Jones has said, I
came across another significant article in the London
Evening Standard of 1975 with the headlines 'Cancer
Charity attacked.' The article goes on to say: 'Misleading
claims over Cancer "cures" and successes in treatment are
being made by the Cancer Research Campaign claimed a
doctor today. This unprecedented attack on the largest
charity organisation raising money for cancer research in
Britain was made in the medical journal "Doctor".

Propaganda and leaflets put out by the campaign exag-
gerated the success rates of treatment, said DR. Louis
Goldman, the medical consultant of the journal.

One advertisement for funds claimed: "When diagnosed
early enough there is now a better than 50 per cent chance
of curing cancer in most parts of the body."

The 'catch' of this particular claim was that many of the
common cancers like lung, stomach and breast, cannot be
diagnosed early.

A leaflet listed 30 cancer sites of tumours and then compared survival rates for three years, when five years was the
more usual period.

"No one who knows anything about cancer therapy or
the way statistics are compiled will accept that the prog-
nosis of cancer of the liver, lungs, breasts, or stomach, to
name only a few has improved significantly in the last
20 years" he says. There were highly selective figures for
breast cancer published too, "The sad fact is that 10,000
of the 16,000 women who develop this disease each year
die from it—almost exactly the same proportion as in the
1940s."

To me this is sufficient indication that things are not as
they seem to be and a lot of forward thinking men from
the medical profession are coming round to think that
giving of drugs, surgery, Xray and Radium therapy is not
the answer to good health. In the last few years between
1970-75 many medical men have come forward and
written books more in line with what has been advocated
by Natural Hygienists and linking health with the pri-
mordial requisites of life namely sound nutrition, adequate
sleep and rest, plenty of exercise, emotional poise coupled
with avoidance of stress factors and fresh air and sunshine.

Notable amongst these Doctors I want to single out, Dr. H. Beiler, MD, author of "Food Is Your Best Medicine", Dr. Alan Cott MD author of "Fasting—The Ultimate Diet", Dr. Andrew Maleison MD author of "Need your Doctor be so useless", Dr. Joan Gomez author of "You need not die young", Dr. J. Cheraskin, author of "Psycho-Dietetics", Dr. J. Lambert Mount M.B.B.S. author of "The health and diet of the western man", Dr. Kenneth Cooper author of "Aerobics", Dr. Alan H. Nittler MD author of "A new breed of Doctor", and Dr. Ivan Illich, author of the book "Medical Nemesis."

They are indeed a new breed of Doctors who have outgrown the idea that health depends on 'drugs' and that the solution of sickness and disease lies not in chemotherapy but in regulating the life style of their patients.

Gentlemen, I salute you for questioning the ancient practice of drug medicine, and for your courage in speaking out the truth as you know it.

CHAPTER XVI

Toxemia Explained

The time to deal with disease is one, two, ten, twenty, fifty years before it appears. But to do this on a large scale we shall have to get rid of medical science first; because by inoculations, immunizations, radium, surgery, x-rays, innumerable poisonous drugs, and incessant cancer, tuberculosis, germ and disease propaganda, it is disseminating and broadcasting disease, preventing recovery and proffering (at a price) an illusory would-be alternative to repentance from wrong living and obedience to the laws or conditions that govern well being.

There will be fervent opposition because as soon as the people wake up to the (still partly unconscious) fraud of medical science, eighty percent of its "services" will not be required—Dr. Ulric Williams, M.B.CHB. (the original "Radio Doctor" in Democracy, N.Z. 15:9:47)

Toxemia and toxins are words commonly used in the Natural Hygiene field, but many people are still in ignorance of what they are and what they imply. In order to understand these two words, it is necessary to understand the function of the body as a whole and also that of each individual cell, of which there are billions and trillions going to form the body.

Now the two main functions of all cells are to nourish themselves by appropriating food from their surroundings and to discard their waste by a process of excretion. When the cells are in full vigor and activity, this process of excretion goes on regularly without any outward symptoms of an obvious nature. As long as the cell has the energy and vitality, its function of nutrition and excretion goes on harmoniously. But as soon as the energy and vitality of the cell or cells is sapped—a process which is called Enervation (and which can be attributed to many causes)—then, like the wheel which has stopped revolving and begins to

211

gather dust, the process of excretion or elimination is suspended or sometimes even completely stopped, and then the accumulation and retention of these waste products takes place in the cell. This is the true constant. This autogenous self-generated poisoning is what we call Toxemia.

Every act of every cell in the body produces waste. This waste is poisonous, i.e. it is incompatible with the life of the cell. Just as the gradual accumulation of alcohol in a mass of fermenting material (e.g. yeast cells) reaches a state of concentration that kills the bacteria that produces the alcohol, so the accumulation of the normal cellular waste in the liquid medium reaches a certain concentration that kills the cells that give it off.

When a piece of human tissue is cultured in a flask, a volume of liquid equal to two thousand times its own volume is required to prevent it from being poisoned in a few days from the accumulation of its own waste—metabolites; Dr. Alexis Carrel, the well known physiologist, proved this time and again. The cells and tissues of the intact organism (e.g. the human body) have the same need for a pure medium but, due to the marvelous ability of the circulatory system in circulating the body's fluids, i.e. the lymph and blood, and of the lungs, liver, and kidneys, with some help from the bowels and skin in excreting the waste, the cells of the body are able to live in a fluid medium of but six to seven quarts. Were the tissues of the average man reduced to small fragments and cultivated in flasks (a la Alexis Carrel's experiments) these would require approximately 52,835 gallons of fluid in which to live. Even then, in time, unless the fluids were changed at intervals, the accumulation of waste would reach a concentration that would kill the tissue fragments. The cells throw their waste into the lymph which carries it back to the blood. The blood takes the waste to the excretory organs mentioned above, for elimination. Normal elimination keeps the blood and lymph clean. Toxemia is hence the aftermath of Enervation.

Enervation, in brief, is the sum total of all our expenditures of nerve energy involved in our day-to-day living. When the sum of our daily expenditures is greater than we can or than we do recuperate daily, we become enervated. When an enervated individual is saturated with toxins, any additional enervating influence that puts an added check to elimination will cause the toxemia to be pushed above the point of toleration, and will precipitate a crisis— a process of compensatory elimination through channels whose main work is not elimination, e.g. the mucous membranes (colds, catarrh, inflammation and skin eruptions.)

Now, what about the word Toxin? Many have asked— but what are the toxins? What is their chemical nature, if any, and where are they in the body if the elimination is poor? We all know that a certain amount of food is needed for the process of nutrition to go on in the living cell. As human beings, we supply this food by what we eat and drink. However, the most wholesome of the food has to be broken down into simpler constituents by the body. Proteins, fats, carbohydrates—all these have to be oxidised to irreducible minimum of carbon dioxide, water, nitrogen, sulphur or phosphorus, which will then pass out of the system being comparatively innocuous. When there is incomplete breakdown of these foods, substances which are highly incompatible with life are formed— known as organic acids (they are pyruvic, lactic, acetic, oxalic, ketoglutaric, succinic, citric, malic, fumaric, etc. acids). The kidneys void urea, uric acid, creatine, creatinine, ammonia, fatty acids, sugar, carbonates and free carbonic acids, etc.—all of which are incompatible with life and must be thrown off.

It must be noted at this point that there is a great structural and functional difference between elimination and voiding. Elimination is the release of toxins from all the tissue cells of the entire body into the blood stream and lymphatic system. It is accomplished by developed differences in the electric polarity of the cell and nuclear membranes, resulting in osmotic pressure changes and cell permeability. These complex electrical phenomena cannot be accelerated by man through any means except by a total physical and physiological rest, allowing the nerve energy to be restored. Voiding is the release from the body of eliminated tissue poisons through the bladder, lungs, skin, and bowels. These latter organs are repositories for the primary poisons ejected by the tissues.

As to where the toxins are:—Natural Hygiene practitioners have pointed out two places where toxins find a resting place. One—the intercellular liquid media, namely the lymph and the connective tissues, together with fat deposits; and two—the bloodstream itself. Recent experiments have proven the validity of this theory. That the human bloodstream is a reservoir of toxic wastes in unhealthy human beings has been the cry of Natural Hygienists, but always denied by the orthodox physicians.

There is, however, an article in Science Magazine, November 1947, by Melvin H. Kinsely and others, captioned "Sludged Blood", which substantiates and confirms this Natural Hygienic theory about the toxicity of the blood. This research covered a period of 16 years and was conducted by a group of physiologists and pathologists. It starts as follows: "This paper constitutes a brief introduction to a series of observations made mostly with microscopes in living animals and men, which leads to a more precise understanding of a variety of mechanisms, whereby injuries and diseases damage the human body. It is felt that these observations clarify a group of fundamental ideas, explain many old experiments, and make the solution simple. The observations also permit, and we think, necessitate a subdivision and reclassification, a much simplified and, for guiding investigations, a more useful classification of many of the currently known pathologic mechanisms of the diseases of animals and men. Our purpose is to present and define certain properties of normal blood, blood flow, and vessel walls; to offer evidence that these properties are necessary to the normal functioning of the circulatory system; to describe certain visible pathogenic structures and processes; and to define goals now necessary for therapeutics."

It goes on to tell of extensive experimentation and how they were able to watch with binocular microscopes the blood as it flowed through the membranes of the eye in both living animals and men. They say further: The circulating red cells not only were not agglutinated (united with glue) but tended to repel each other slightly. In carefully handled tissues, red cell rouleaux (rolls of cells resembling piles of coins) were not present. The normal red blood cells were not coated with any microscopically visible protein precipitate. The fact that they show no tendency to adhere to each other in view is evidence that they are not coated with any very thin, transparent, or oherwise invisible sticky precipitate. These observations are in strict agreement with those of many previous investigations. No white cells or erythrocytes (red cells) stuck to the inner surfaces of the walls of small vessels. The inner surfaces of the linings of normal vessels were smooth and clean". "The flow of the unagglutinated blood was laminar or streamlined." "In small arteries and veins the blood cells were in an axial stream and around them was a peripheral concentric layer of plasma. The cells of the stream were arranged in concentric laminae, the center one passing along most rapidly, and each additional layer passing more slowly than the one inside it. The wall of each lamina of this system consisted of unagglutinated blood cells; each layer was exactly one red cell thick (film recorded)."

"This arrangement of unagglutinated blood cells in fluid plasma is a necessary part of the highest degree of good health, as the next succeeding paragraphs show. The rates of flow of blood through each tissue of each organ of the body set the maximum rate at which the cells of that tissue can receive blood-born materials. For this discussion the most important of these is oxygen; it is necessary to all cells of the body; it is not stored in the body, and even slight local oxygen deficits are known to begin to upset many factors of physiology." They describe healthy, normal blood, its rate of flow, and they also describe blood vessel walls. They say that no blood seeped through the vessel walls. Continuing, they say: "In about 600 unanaesthetised human patients, diagnosed by practising physicians as having a wide variety of pathologic conditions and diseases, we have seen the blood cells agglutinated into masses (not rouleaux); this changed the blood from its normal, relatively fluid state, to a circulating sludge."

Then follows a list of more than 50 diseases which afflicted the above-mentioned patients. It was found then that "all these people had sludged blood." Also that in 23 pregnancies which had pathologic complications, 22 had sludged blood. Again I quote: "Thus far, completely unagglutinated blood has been found only in strictly healthy animals and men. Mild degrees of intravascular agglutination have been seen in many laboratory workers, students and colleagues in the Chicago area where sinusitis of various degrees of severity and other afflictions of the upper respiratory system are endemic. The more severe degrees of intravascular agglutination have been exhibited only in animals during controlled experiments and in persons who were sufficiently ill to have placed themselves under the care of physicians. No severely ill person has yet been seen who did not have intravascular agglutination of the blood and visibly pathologic vessel walls." There are several more pages, but the preceeding covers the most important part.

To summarise: they found in ill people and animals that the blood was thick, flowed slowly, and seeped through the vessel walls. None of the conditions occurred in healthy people. Hygienists from the earliest writers to the present ones have maintained that this sludging, or thickening, does occur in the blood. So all these investigations merely corroborate and prove what Hygienists have taught for more than a century. Despite all this knowledge now in the hands of the medical profession, it is of little value to them because they do not know the cause of these abnormal conditions.

Natural Hygienists know the cause, and they also know how to remove it. Fasting will enable the body to rid itself of toxins, and Hygienic living will prevent their re-occurrence.

CHAPTER XVII

A New Concept of Health

Health is not only absence of illness:—
It is the deep longing of the whole
Noiselessly yet irresistably traveling to its goal.

Health is not only bulging muscles:—
It is the symmetry of mind and body;
The men sanna in corpo sanno;
A remembrance of the Golden Age.

Health is not only absence of death:—
It is life, the "joie de vivre"
Welling up soundlessly, yet with that urge
That brings to beauty the simpler things
Enfolding us with joy too deep for words.

Health is the cessation of struggle;
The absence of fear
The emptying of bad habits;
The upsurge of the whole into holiness;
And out of such health, springs true creation.

Health is not loneliness:—
It is the deep companionship of every organ,
Functioning in unison too rare for belief.

(From "Words and Music and All Alone"
by K. R. Sidhwa)

Why should anyone want to know anything about the human being, his body, and his mind? And for that matter, why should anyone believe that knowledge of the human mind and body is either unobtainable or undesirable? Why should men ostensibly seeking an answer to the suffering of human beings, stray so far from it as to examine rats and guinea pigs, and entirely avoid looking at human beings and their mode of living? And why should anyone pretending to help towards recovery of health, stray so far afield as electric shock, artificial fevers and poisonous drugs?

The answers are relatively simple. Anyone who knows the structure, function, and dynamics of the human mind-body entity knows it is very difficult to control. The only way a person's attitude is controlled is by enforcing upon him ignorance of himself.

As far as study and recovery are concerned, a human being who has been made ignorant of his mind-body entity, would have to have restored to him awareness of himself fundamentally, before he could be considered to be progressing towards recovery. And when one restores full awareness to the human being, it is likely that one is no longer able to victimize it. And a profession or a society would have to move out of slave orientation into action by freedom and consent, were it to be effective.

Just as you do not want people to control you, so you should want knowledge of yourself. Just as you fight away from knowingness concerning self, so you will be controlled.

A simple and conclusive science of mind-body is a vital necessity in any society which would combat or contest or dispute, and effort to attain such a science would be those interests which desire, by ignorance or willfulness, to maintain their control of slavery. Each and every impulse of freedom is an impulse towards sanity, towards health, towards happiness. Every impulse towards slavery is an impulse in the direction of misery, disease, and death. One can say alike of the arthritic and the neurotic that the basic cause of disturbance, physical or mental, is germinated in efforts to reduce the freedom of the individual, the group or mankind, from being aware of his individual mode of life.

Natural Hygiene is therefore that effort towards the attainment by man of a level of freedom where decency and happiness can prevail, and where knowledge of health, disease and healing would prevent the unscrupulous use of the mechanisms of slavery. Natural Hygiene can be contested, it can be vilified, its founders and practitioners can be publicly pilloried, but Natural Hygiene cannot be ignored. It could neither be drowned in praise nor burned in some purge to its total irradication, for it is a praiseworthy observable fact that the one impulse in man which cannot be erased is his impulse towards freedom, his impulse towards sanity, towards a higher level of attainment in all of his endeavors. This is man's one saving grace, and because Natural Hygiene is such an impulse, and because its basic purpose is so fundamental from the moment of its conception, and has been dedicated unswervably to the attainment of even greater freedom, it cannot perish. This is a fact which will become doubtlessly more annoying to the slave masters, the treatment mongers, and peddlers of "cure-all" modalities, as the years roll on.

There is more argument upon which we could adventure concerning whether Natural Hygiene is an art or a science, whether it a humanity or a hoax, but all these would avail us very little for we would only be quibbling with words. Natural Hygiene is what it is, and the totality of it can best be summed by the description "an understanding of man." We do not care whether it can be called an art or a science or both. We do not care whether or not it is more properly catalogued under adventure or mystery. We do care whether or not it is promulgated and known, for everywhere it walks, slavery ceases. That mind-body which understands itself is the free man. He is no longer prone to obsessive behavior, unthinking, compliances, cowardly innuendoes. He is at home in his natural environment, not a stranger. By learning to understand disease and ill-health, he is free to proceed towards health, which is his birthright. He no longer fears "catching diseases," but he is mindful of the fact, that any catching that is to be done by him is to catch himself napping as regards his mode of living, and his various habits in eating, drinking, sleeping, resting, exercising, etc., which lead him to enervation.

Why should you as a person know something about your health or lack of it? A question of a similar magnitude would be "why should you live?" A writer of science fiction once conceived a world composed entirely of machines, composed to a point where the machines were repaired by other machines, which in turn were repaired by other machines, and so the circle went round and the machine survived. He wrote this story from the fondest belief of nuclear physics that there is only a machine, that man derives from some spontaneous combustion of some chemicals in the laboratory, that freedom is impossible, that all behavior is stimulus-response, that causative thought cannot exist. What a world this would be! And yet this world, this pattern, is the goal of the slave-makers. If every man could be depressed from his freedom to a point where he believed himself but the cog in an enormous machine, then all things would be enslaved. Hence the present day official idea that disease and ill health are part and parcel of a man's life, depending on chance and circumstances outside his own control and domain, where war, pestilence and disease are as inevitable as the rising of the sun, is promulgated to entrap the unsuspecting individual in the vicious circle, which can only be broken into if one has the means to pacify the greed of the so-called soothsayers, cure-mongers, and dope peddlers.

Thus as we depart from the concepts of freedom, we depart into a darkness where the will, the fear, or the brutality of one or a few, no matter how well educated, may yet obliterate everything for which we have worked, everything for which we have hoped, in human health and happiness. This is what happens when the machine runs wild and when man, becoming a machine, runs wild. Man can only become a machine when he is no longer capable of understanding his own beingness and has lost his contact with it. Hence it is of utmost urgency that each of us understand something about our mind-body entity, that we understand that we are thinking human beings and not robots, and it is of great value that man attain at once an insight into his capacity for freedom, where the machine reaction of destruction may be controlled, and where man himself can enjoy some of the happiness to which he is entitled.

For most of us who have problems, the difficulty lies in that we try to solve each problem on its own plane. We do not try to solve the problem as a whole, but try to solve it from a particular point of view, or we try to differentiate, or separate, the problem from the total process, which is life. If we have an economic problem, we try to solve it on that plane alone, disregarding the total process of life; and each problem when so tackled, obviously must fail to be solved; because our life is not in water-tight compartments. Our life is a total process, psychologically as well as physiologically, and when we try to solve the psychological problems without understanding the physiological problems, we give wrong emphasis and therefore further complicate the problem.

What we have to do, it seems to us, is to take each problem and not deal with it as a separate issue, but as part of a whole.

If we take such an approach to our problems, we shall be able to understand, not only the problems, but the whole significance of our existence. Now what do we mean by a problem? Surely we mean a state in which there is conflict. As long as there is conflict in us, we regard that conflict as a problem, as something to be dissolved, to be understood, or from which we wish to escape. So we approach a problem, a conflict, do we not, either desiring to escape from it or to find an answer for it, to find a solution for it.

Now please think: is the solution different from the problem, or does the solution lie in understanding the problem itself, and not away from it? Obviously those of us who want to escape from a problem have innumerable ways—drinks, drugs, narcotics, amusements, religious or psychological illusions, and so on. It is comparatively easy to find an escape from our problems and shut our eyes to them, which most of us do, because we do not know how to tackle them. We always have ready-made answers according to our beliefs, our prejudices, according to what a teacher, a doctor, or our parents have told us, and with that ready-made answer we try to solve, to approach the problem. Surely that doesn't solve it; that is but another form of escape.

So it seems to us that to understand a problem requires not a ready-made answer, not trying to seek a solution for the problem, but a direct consideration of the problem itself, which is to approach it without the desire to find an answer, if one may so put it. Then you are directly in relationship with the problem, then you are the problem, i.e. the problem is no longer separate from yourself. And we think that is the first thing we must realize, that the problem of existence, with all its complexities, is not different from ourselves. We are the problem, and as long as we regard the problem as something away from us, or apart from us, our approach must inevitably end in failure. Whereas if we regard the problem as our own, as part of us, then perhaps we can begin to understand it significantly —which means, essentially, does it not, that a problem exists because there is no self-knowledge.

So it seems to us, our difficulty in understanding the many problems that confront us comes about through ignorance of ourselves. It is we who create the problem, we who are part of the environment as well as something more. Now you may well ask, what has all this to do with "health"? Where does "curing" of disease come in? Well, isn't it a fact that you are reading this book because you are worried, anxious, apprehensive and panicky about your lack of health, i.e. you have a health problem?

And why have you a health problem? Because you have refused to see the problem, to understand the whys and wherefores of the functions of your own body, because being conditioned from childhood with various beliefs, prejudices, with so-called authoritative statements, you have looked upon various ailments and sufferings as a dispensation of so-called Divine Providence. It is nothing of the sort! As Dr. Tilden, one of the greatest pioneers of Natural Hygiene, puts it, "disease is a dispensation of damned ignorance rather than Divine Providence." Most of you have tried various means of escape, in trying to run away from disease, in trying to solve this vital problem of health and disease by various means—drugs, injections, herbs, pills, powders, charms and amulets and all so-called remedies; you have refused to face the problem.

Now therefore, let us together face this problem and in doing so, discover for ourselves the so-called mystery of maintaining good health. So now what is Natural Hygiene? Many of you, like millions of others, are ignorant about it. To some it has meant eating of grass and apples, to others a perpetual stewing or freezing in water, to others running about naked, and to many more just the plain simple words "of course, vegetarianism."

All of these people have sincerely believed that their conception of Natural Hygiene is true, with the result they have shied away from the opportunity of a solution to their many problems. For Natural Hygiene in its broadest sense is an investigation, an attempt to face reality, the facts governing the structure and function of our living bodies.

Hence the need for understanding the Basic Principles

in Natural Hygiene. What are they? The three principles of utmost importance that come to mind are:

(1) That the body contains within itself the supreme Intelligence and power to heal itself, e.g. a wound.

(2) That good health is rarely placid, i.e. a body in vigorous health throws out, or tries to throw out, any toxins which are forced upon it. And last but no least,

(3) The famous phrase of Dr. Louis Kuhne "there is but one disease—tissue uncleanliness", or what we Hygienists term as Toxemia in Natural Hygiene.

To some of you this may sound all new and fascinating, but was there ever a discovery that was not novel, or a truth that was not astounding to somebody? Now let us deal briefly with each of these sub-titles.

The first point is missed not only by lay people but by the average professional physician, practising medicine. The most important thing to remember here is that, provided the body is left *"intelligently alone"*, it will progress towards recovery and healing, and we have ourselves witnessed personally many such cases where the body has done an amazing job after a negative pronouncement by the medical profession. But how many stop to think whether the body will be much better off without their various aids and remedies, which they think they are giving?

Many times we have been told by some of our patients, "Yes, I have been doing exactly what you have asked me to do, but I am not getting any better;" then on questioning they come out with this burst, "Yes, I have been taking this thing and doing that thing plus all you said, because I thought it would help me to get better quickly." Help the body? Help Nature? We know that no one can help Nature to do her own job—whatever we Natural Hygiene practitioners do is to teach the patient to stop interfering with the body and help him remove obstruction from Nature's path so that she can carry on the job unhindered.

As regards the second point, many people ask us, "What is our attitude towards so-called acute diseases, for example, a cold or fever?" The answer is that Natural Hygiene does not look upon acute disease as something to be afraid of, something to fight against, as do the orthodox medical practitioners. Natural Hygiene looks upon acute disease as a process of purification which helps the body to gain a firm foothold towards health, provided the body is allowed to do its job as it was meant to do. Natural Hygiene looks upon acute disease as an effort on the part of the body to get rid of the accumulated toxins and waste products, which have been allowed to collect in the system, due to unhealthy habits on the part of that individual. People mistake healthy reactions for disease and try to stop them. Indeed, except for the Natural Hygiene school, health as such is not investigated. The usual acceptance is that health is a negative quality—a mere absence of the symptoms of disease. This conception is ludicrously false. Instead, the symptoms of disease shows off the vitality of the body to cope with the accumulative effects of various abuses on the body, and the disease process as an emergency attempt to clean the system.

When people will look upon diseases as "healing crises" and regard them as such, instead of thwarting their efforts with drugs, injections and eating plenty to "keep up their strength", then Natural Hygiene will have scored one more goal towards a new concept of healthy living.

As regards the third point, the fallacy of symptomatic treatment has been amply pointed out in previous pages. Natural Hygiene does not neglect the increased knowledge of the body—neither does it deny the existence of microbes called disease germs. But it teaches that these microbes do not start the trouble. They appear and flourish only where there is sufficient matter for them to feed on, and they cannot feed on healthy living tissue, but only on broken down and toxic matter, and as such, these microbes are really the life savers in a certain way as they warn us by their breeding that there is accumulated waste in our tissues, and we should be doing something about it.

Today the word disease is largely abused, thanks to the medical profession; one wonders as to how many of you reading this book have the correct meaning of the word disease. How many of you still believe that disease is an entity by itself, that it is a certain thing with its own peculiar properties, which attacks us or is seated within us, or sweeps the country like a fire, etc.? These expressions are not mere metaphors—but express the age-old ideas and superstitious theories that diseases are substances outside the organic domain. To talk of banishing a disease or wiping it out, or conquering it, is to talk of disease as if it were an evil spirit from some other world, which has penetrated your body. Even the most modern medical ideas have harbored this "evil spirit" superstition, except for the spirit we have now all kinds of germs and viruses as an entity, invading the body instead of the "evil spirit". Now anyone practising unorthodox methods of "caring for the sick" outside the medical profession is termed a quack or a charlatan by that august body; but we agree with Sir Sidney Smith, who says that "the principal cause of quackery outside the medical profession is the quackery going on in the medical profession itself." Disease simply means dis-ease or un-ease, dis-comfort, lack of ease. Sitting on a bed of nails may produce a discom-fort, dis-ease, but the nails are not evil, nor is the pain produced. Disease is essentially a vital action. Let me quote a statement from Dr. Shelton, "In relation between lifeless and living matter, all action is on the side of the vital organism and none whatever on the part of the lifeless object."

Yes, disease may be termed as an attack, but it is not an attack upon the body from without; it is an attack by the body upon morbific agents within, i.e. toxins. We must understand this important concept, that this "vital action" which the body undergoes is the disease. That it is not something which has to be removed or cured. All vital activities, whether they may be disease or health, are carried on under the law of self-preservation.

If we are sick, this is because it is best for us to be sick, i.e. to say, that there are occasions in life in which your getting sick is the only possible way for your body to correct these conditions. Deprive a living body of its ability to manifest its repugnance to incompatible things, in the defensive manner we call morbid action or disease, and you deprive it of life itself. Disease is therefore a product of life. Disease as such is never seen in the dead. But please do not think that we like people to have diseases and that they are necessary.

Disease is an expensive action. Every elimination of even the least virulent toxins by the body, e.g. colds, fever, boils, create a certain amount of strain on the potential vitality of the body. Disease uses up this vital force. But if people live in harmony with the laws of right food, drink, sleep, etc., there is no reason why people should have diseases; only transgressions bring about sickness and misery. Drugs are therefore suppressive. They are able to mask the symptoms, until the body has dealt with the drug, and is vital enough again to take on the cleansing job, from which it was diverted by taking the drugs.

You may well ask—if disease is a remedial process or an effort at getting well, why do not all sick people get well? The answer to this is that it depends on the vitality of the body, on the amount of damage done, and the continuance of the factors that have brought about this effort.

The remedial action of disease is not always successful in accomplishing its purpose because the occasions are far too great for that action to remove. The vitality of that body, after years of effort or resistance against the abuses piled on it, has reached a stage where it can only do a certain amount of mending and healing. The people who do not get well are, in the majority of cases, those people who have continued the abusive habits against the body, in spite of its many warnings, or those who have stifled those warnings with improper or symptomatic treatment, until the body eventually gives up all attempts at restoration, decays, and dies.

Remember that the mill cannot grind with the water that has passed, nor can life be maintained with power that has already been spent.

Anyhow, Natural Hygiene deals with individuals and does not make a generalized statement about specific symptoms. This fact has often to be registered in our patients' minds before we begin to get the desired results. Often we come across cases where two people are supposed to have identical symptoms, as diagnosed in the orthodox way. One showed improvement in a matter of days or weeks, and the other has still to plod on for months or years, husbanding his or her vitality. Then there are patients who ask, "How long have I to follow your instructions?" and always our answer is, "until you are tired of living a healthy and long life," and this answer often brings back a look of surprise and dejection on their faces. They are the ones who do not realize that the things which we have asked them to do and not to do, for getting better, also help them to be alive and on their feet. They do not realize that it is their own responsibility to be healthy as well as alive. They do not see the connection between their present state of ill-health and their previous unhealthy mode of living, which they have been asked to alter in order to get well. On the face of it, they have the impertinence to ask, when can they start all their bad habits again and still continue to remain in good health.

No doubt Dr. Alexander Bryce once said, "Nothing offends patients more than to interfere with their habits of life; their desire is to break every known law of nature, and when they get sick they accept complete absolution in a bottle or two of medicine—they merely want to be patched up sufficiently so they can go right back to their former habits of self-indulgence in its various forms."

People must realize the connection between the cause and the effect, their daily habits and their health, their thoughts and their deeds. That the "cure" of ill-health lies in their hands and it is their sole responsibility, if they want to get well or otherwise. Such is the attitude of mind that is being fostered by the medical profession and, sorry to say, the clergy as well. The charitable grave kindly draws the mantle of oblivion over the victim of such delusions while the priest, pointing to a happier post-mortem existence above the clouds, "soothes the dull, cold ear of death," and thus ignorance flourishes age after age. The clergy has always covered up for the medical profession after their treatment has killed a patient. The clergymen would preach the funeral oration and explain that "God, in His mercy, had removed the deceased." If ever there was such a thing as blasphemy or sacrilege, this is it. To blame God for all the deaths committed by folly of ignorant men. After all, Nature does not work in this way. It does not bribe us to sin by promising us absolution. But the drug peddlers and pill vendors do. They promise us that we can eat what we like, drink what we like, commit nerve-destroying excesses, and transgress all the rules of sane Hygiene, and all will be forgiven if we just take their red, white and blue powders from two to twenty times a day.

No doubt the average man brought up amongst such beliefs and dogmas thinks in the terms of "Why be good when you can buy a "cure"? This type of thinking not only leads to physical degeneration and deterioration, but is most demoralizing too. Natural Hygiene, on the other hand, throws back the responsibility on their own shoulders, and thus prepares them for that inner discipline, which is the only correct answer.

This remedy mentality is so ingrained in us, through mass propaganda of commercial monopolies, that even those who should know better fall for such tempting baits of many phoney dietitians who have sprung up recently, to cash in on the pioneering work of Natural Hygiene.

People must learn to banish from their minds this idea of a specific cure for a specific disease—they must learn to look upon the body as a whole combined unit.

Has it ever occurred to these people that when following their grape diet or rice diet, they have most probably stopped doing many of the silly indiscretions that were keeping them sick, and that it was by giving the body a physiological rest that they have overcome their ailments, and that it was not the grapes or rice that did it? You will see if you will experiment with this—and it will not take a long period of time. But you must give your whole attention, your whole interest to it. And I am not at all sure that most of us do not like to be confused—because in the state of confusion you need not act, and so we are satisfied with confusion; because to understand confusion, chaos, whether in the body or mind, demands action, which is unlike the pursuit of wishful thinking. It is imperative that we investigate this matter fully; for ignorance breeds fear.

One half of the world is drugged to death when sick, and one half of the remainder is fretted and frightened to death. As for the question which so often arises, "What do we substitute then for drugs?", we do not have to choose between two evils.

We must reject them all and choose healthful materials and agencies, and learn to respect ourselves and our body and take sensible care of it. Do that, then watch and wait. For waiting, with that passive awareness and alert watchfulness, is as necessary as doing.

Remember that tall oaks from little acorns grow, and huge streams may flow from small fountains, but fatal diseases do not arise from trifling causes.

Natural Hygiene is not to be looked upon as just a form of therapeutics, whose benefit you can take when you are not feeling up to the mark. It should not be looked upon as a palliative, or tonic, to help you jog along for a few years more on the pathway of life. It should be something which should form a comprehensive unit in the cycle of your life—you should not only practise Natural Hygiene on off days, like Sunday churchgoing, but live Natural Hygiene; mold it not in flesh and bones, as health and fitness, but also create it within your thoughts and deeds. The name Natural Hygiene does not matter a great deal as long as you live it. It will throw out its own radiance wherever you go.

To those of you who are in the Natural Hygiene movement, it represents not only a philosophy of living but also a blueprint by which we can bring realization to that philosophy. Natural Hygiene is a complete way of life, in that its influence is felt in every phase—the physical, the moral, the aesthetic, and regrettably the economic, if we may add a touch of irony. On the physical side it offers us genuine health. On the moral side it offers us lasting hope. On the aesthetic side it offers us true happiness.

We are not Utopians. We are not unrealistic searchers for the unattainable. We are not impracticable dreamers. We are forced to walk alone sometimes, but we are not aloof to the related needs of man in community. We look upon Natural Hygiene as an investment in the future, an opportunity to ease the burdens of the present, and as a means of clarifying the past. The preservation of health and attainment of longevity are not the only motives that influence the Natural Hygiene movement. We do say, however, that they are basic to all else.

Health of mind and body is essential to moral and social health; it is essential to industrial efficiency and to just rulership.

The pursuit of health is therefore not inconsistent with the pursuit of virtue and goodness, but an important part of such pursuit. Health of man is the health of the whole man—it is wholeness, integrity.

With Herophilus (physician to Alexander the Great) we repeat that "When health is absent, wisdom cannot reveal itself, art cannot become manifest, strength cannot fight, wealth becomes useless, and intelligence cannot be applied." To those of you who have been reared on a diet of processed foods, processed thoughts, and processed hopes in the search of one "cure" after another, we hope to show you how re-education of a person's mode of life and living can help him to recovery and health. "Man's history" as H. G. Wells says, "is a race between education and catastrophe." The race must be won by education, and the Natural Hygiene movement is trying its utmost to further that ideal.

Summing up therefore, Natural Hygiene asserts that the world's redemption from disease, drugs and discord depends on a practical recognition—that nature's laws cannot be violated with impunity; that penalties will not be remitted; that nature has not provided so-called remedies; that if wrong is done, evil consquences will follow; that every poisonous drug and every unphysiological habit and every unhealthful act will make its injurious mark irrevocably and forever; that our life, our strength, our health will be measured by our observances of organic law. This is a statement of vital truth, the full realization of which, by the people as a whole, will lead inevitably to a revolution in their various modes of living. For the beginning of Natural Hygiene philosophy is to "cease to do evil"—it will be easy thereafter to "learn to do good." In the East there is a saying "The journey of a thousand miles starts with one step," and your journey today to the kingdom of health will start with that first step—your conception of what health means to you. Choose your own compensation and thereby choose your own course.

CHAPTER XVIII

What Natural Hygiene is up Against

"Only that which is whole is Truth"
(Hegel)—German Philosopher

Empty handed and alone I entered this World,
Rich with life and alone I wandered all my days.
My wanderings are done now, life spent, yet still
  alone.
I journey back, spacing my days,
For the home-coming that will be mine.
(From "Words and Music and All Alone"
by K. R. SIDHWA)

Often we have been asked by sincere folks all over the world: "If Natural Hygiene is what you say it is, and if it is an open door to health and happiness, why is it not popular, and why do governments of different nations ignore it?" To brush the question aside with a shrug and dismiss it by saying "vested interests", "commercialism' is not enough. People must know as much as possible about how the dice are loaded against Natural Hygiene and its practitioners.

To apply the principles and practices of Natural Hygiene is gradually becoming more and more difficult in a so-called civilized world. Let us imagine the life of a baby born to Mr. and Mrs. Average. Observe the numerous obstacles he will have to hurdle. First of all, an average civilized mother will refuse to breast-feed the baby, and many more will not be able to do so. Then there will be the difficulty of obtaining fresh, clean, unpasteurized, unadulterated milk. In many countries (except in the villages) the milk industry has so ordained it that pasteurized milk is actually cheaper in price than the fresh unpasteurized variety. Since city life is the accepted feature of modern-day living, most babies will be born in an atmosphere polluted by soot, smog, diesel and petrol fumes and will have to live in sulphur-laden air. In most countries poverty is still rife, with overcrowding, slums, unsatisfactory sanitary arrangements, and an inadequate clean water supply. Hence, most babies will have to combat such unhealthy surroundings.

Then, as though adding insult to injury, the city authorities will urge the parents to have their child injected with drugs, immunized and vaccinated—a mean substitute for what should be their birthright. Fear of disease and glorification of the orthodox medical doctor will be gradually instilled in the child. As soon as he has reached the weaning stage, all sorts of proprietary brand foods, containing as much real food value as the tins and packets they come in, will be thrust upon him by the ignorant and unsuspecting parents, in the belief that anything that is devised in the laboratory is superior to nature's own bounty. Thus the senses of the child are perverted from the very beginning.

Apart from the ignorant and sometimes foolish sophisticated parents who habituate the child to modern dietetic practice, the relatives and friends will push one more nail into his already depleted energy by insisting on keeping him awake into the late hours of the night and stimulating his imagination and appetite by excitement and candy. But this is not enough. By example and precept they condition the child to accept narcotics, tea, coffee, alcohol, soft drinks and smoking as normal practices, and to believe that disease is something we all have to put up with, as if there is a place for a so-called necessary evil. As soon as they are able to toddle on their feet, they are packed off to school to be burdened with untimely responsibilities in the form of excess study and homework so that they are children no more, but little adults with their own fears, phobias and tensions.

It is a miracle that most of them survive! Soon their little minds and bodies begin to protest against their civilized treatment, and their doom is sealed. The cure-mongers and treatment-peddlers move in en masse, backed by chemical cartels, drug industries, and various gadget makers. Prescriptions will flow in a steady stream until their little insides are pickled with proprietary poisons. As soon as the child emerges half-dead from such procedures, now grown into adolescence, he comes into contact with the "come hither" signs of all sorts of advertisements—in books, magazines, on film, on television, on billboards, etc.—with all who are out to extract from him the little pocket money he may have. With such an example of a ruthless, competitive world where evil prevails and truth is trodden down, what sort of moral health can the child inherit? Dr. Shelton is very optimistic, claiming that the Natural Hygiene millenium will arrive. We hope he is right. The situation is still grim, in our opinion.

Now supposing the child has arrived at his adulthood, and suppose by chance he has come in contact with Natural Hygiene, can you imagine the terrible conflicts he has to undergo? To doubt his whole upbringing—his parents, teachers, friends and the society about him. He suddenly finds that he is not "with it." It takes tremendous courage, patience, determination and the will to serve, to stick to the new discovery he has made. At every step he is spurned, rejected, laughed at, ridiculed, and made to doubt his very existence. He finds it difficult to get a mate, and his spirit and fun out of life are dampened. No doubt many fall by the wayside.

Apart from the vested and commercial interests of the drug industry, the other interests sided against Natural Hygiene are as follows:

(1) The chemical fertilizers, insecticides and pesticides manufactured, so that organically grown food becomes expensive and sometimes way beyond the reach of an average income.

(2) The alcohol and spirit industries and the great breweries.

(3) The butchers and the meat, fish and poultry trade.

(4) The millers and makers of white flour and its by-products.

(5) The tobacco industry.

(6) The cosmetic industry.

(7) The dentists, doctors and deans of medical colleges.

(8) The spice and salt merchants.

(9) The water polluters with their fluorides and chlorides.

(10) The sugar refineries and their by-products.

(11) Tea, coffee, and cocoa-bean planters.

(12) The druggist, chemist and all those who sell their products.

(13) Hoteliers and restaurant owners and their army of chefs and sub-chefs who are expert in the art of concocting foodless food with their sense-perverting aromas and flavors.

(14) The nursing profession who under a hygienic way of life would have to do more nursing than fussing and doling out drugs on behalf of the medical doctors.

(15) All the so-called schools of healing, which whilst paying lip-service to vis meditrix naturae, will do anything to prevent their clients from going to a Natural Hygiene institution. We have had bitter experiences. Our patients were told "They are too radical, they are very strict. Fasting will kill you. Treatment, colonic irrigations, herbs, homeopathic medicines are all necessary to cleanse your system. We will allow a compromise—you can smoke, drink, have tea, coffee, cakes and sweets in moderation. There is no need to give up flesh, fish or fowl. Salt and spices bring zest to your appetite and stimulate gastric digestion—have them in moderation."

Now we can understand why no government will recognize Natural Hygiene in toto. All governments are governed, not by the people, but by vested interests of big industries which finance the governments. Certain allowances will be made to lull us into a false sense of security. Certain aspects of Hygiene will be recognized, but no government is going to antagonise the above-named industries and their by-products. It will not be safe. Besides all these, in many parts of the world very few have the time and energy to obtain sufficient sleep, relaxation and exercise. Overworking mentally and physically, many have not really the time. Our socio-economic structure is such that not all have enough leisure hours, or if they have, they do not know how to utilize them.

We know of one individual at least who just could not take time off for a long fast which he needed badly in order to overcome a chronic ailment. Circumstances were such that one way or another he had to continue to be on his feet in order to keep a large family going. His only solution was to be subsidized for such a period of rest.

These are the reasons why we say that Natural Hygiene is not only a reformative movement but a revolutionary one—the whole existing pattern of life needs to be changed if humanity at large is to live Hygienically.

Let us endeavor in the hope that in spite of such odds, Natural Hygiene will ultimately be accepted.

INDEX

237

NATURAL HYGIENE PRESS
BOOK ORDER FORM U

- [ ] A—FASTING CAN SAVE YOUR LIFE $1.75
- [ ] B—YOU DON'T HAVE TO BE SICK! $1.45
- [ ] C—HEALTH FOR THE MILLIONS $1.45
- [ ] D—HYGIENIC CARE OF CHILDREN $1.95
- [ ] E—EXERCISE! $1.95
- [ ] F—THE GREATEST HEALTH DISCOVERY $1.75
- [ ] G—DICTIONARY OF MAN'S FOOD $2.25
- [ ] H—TOXEMIA $1.50
- [ ] I—PROGRAM FOR DYNAMIC HEALTH $1.00
- [ ] J—FASTING FOR RENEWAL OF LIFE $2.25
- [ ] K—DON'T GET STUCK—VIA VACCINATIONS AND INJECTIONS $2.00
- [ ] L—SUPERIOR FOODS, DIET PRINCIPLES AND PRACTICES, ETC. $1.50
- [ ] M—THE HAPPY TRUTH ABOUT PROTEIN $1.00
- [ ] N—DIAGNOSIS CANCER—ESCAPE FEAR VIA NATURAL HYGIENE $1.00
- [ ] O—PLEASE DON'T SMOKE IN OUR HOUSE $1.50
- [ ] P—FOODS FOR PLEASURE & HEALTH; HANDBOOK FOR HYGIENIC LIVING $2.50
- [ ] Q—FOOD COMBINING MADE EASY $1.50
- [ ] R—SUPERIOR NUTRITION $3.25
- [ ] T—FIT FOOD FOR MAN   .50
- [ ] U—MEDICAL DRUGS ON TRIAL $2.25
- [ ] JA—THE HYGIENIC SYSTEM, VOL. I $5.00
- [ ] JB—SYPHILIS: THE WEREWOLF OF MEDICINE $4.50
- [ ] JC—LIVING LIFE TO LIVE IT LONGER $3.00
- [ ] JD—FASTING FOR HEALTH AND LONG LIFE $3.00
- [ ] JE—AN INTRODUCTION TO NATURAL HYGIENE $2.00
- [ ] JF—THERAPEUTIC FASTING $2.50
- [ ] XA—THE HYGIENIC SYSTEM, VOL. II—COMPLETE GUIDE TO FOOD AND FEEDING $7.50
- [ ] XC—NATURAL HYGIENE: MAN'S PRISTINE WAY OF LIFE $7.50
- [ ] XD—HUMAN BEAUTY: ITS CULTURE AND HYGIENE $12.50
- [ ] XF—CORRECT FOOD COMBINING PLACE MAT (PLUS 45¢ P&H) $1.50
- [ ] XH—A GIFT OF LOVE $7.50
- [ ] DR. SHELTON'S HYGIENIC REVIEW $7.50/YR.
  ($8/YR. Canada, Foreign)

● ADD 25¢ TO EACH BOOK FOR POSTAGE AND HANDLING CHARGES.

● SEE NEXT PAGE FOR ORDER BLANK

TOTAL $_____

NOTICE TO THE READER

If after reading this book, you feel the vital knowledge which it contains deserves to be made widely known, you are urged to become a member of the American Natural Hygiene Society and help to contribute to this worthy cause for the benefit of mankind. (Contributions, wills, bequests are tax exempt.)

As a membership bonus we will send this book or any other N.H.P. publication in value up to $1.95 to anyone of your choice. Fill out the application below and mail your remittance of $11.00 for your membership and the bonus book. Outside U.S.A.—$12.00.

☐—Please enroll me as a member of your worthy cause. Enclosed find $11.00 *payable in U. S. $ to A.N.H.S.* for the annual *membership and bonus book.*

☐—BOOK ORDER—Enclosed find $_____for books indicated on order form "U" Payable in U. S. $ to NATURAL HYGIENE PRESS.

Name_____
(please print)

Address_____

City, State, Zip_____

Phone No._____Age_____

SEND BONUS BOOK TITLED_____

_____

To_____
(please print)

Address_____

City, State, Zip_____

AMERICAN NATURAL HYGIENE SOCIETY, Dept U.
1920 IRVING PARK ROAD, CHICAGO, ILL. 60613

U

HIISTORICAL BACKGROUND

Natural Hygiene Press, the publisher of this book, is a division of the American Natural Hygiene Society. The Society is a non-profit, tax exempt membership organization founded in 1949 for the primary purpose of public education in *Natural Hygiene,* which is a system, based on biology and physiology, for preserving and recovering health through natural living habits.

Natural Hygiene came on the American scene as an educational movement in 1830 through the lectures of Sylvester Graham in New York, Rochester, Providence, Buffalo and other eastern cities. Modern dietary science is said to have had its beginning with Graham, who stressed the value of fresh fruits and vegetables as the best foods for man. He wrote books and articles on healthful living for 21 years and his greatest work is the *Science of Human Life,* published in 1839.

Graham pioneered in this country in advocating the teaching of physiology in the public schools and in expounding the value of regular physical exercise, fresh air and well ventilated homes, rest and sleep, sunbathing, emotional control and clothing reform for women from the tight waists, corsets and high heeled pointed toed shoes of the day.

Graham was joined in his work of health education by prominent medical people of the time such as Isaac Jennings, M.D., William Alcott, M.D., Russell Thacker Trall, M.D., Thomas Low Nichols, M.D., Susanna Dodds, M.D., James Caleb Jackson, M.D., George H. Taylor, M.D., and later by Robert Walker, M.D., John H. Tilden, M.D.

Many of these pioneers of the *Natural Hygiene* System had suffered serious illness during their early years which became a strong motivating force in seeking the solution to the disease problem. They came to see in wrong living the true cause of disease and sought to induce mankind to return to a normal way of life by adopting good living habits. They wrote prodigiously in books and magazines and some founded colleges to train students in caring for people through hygienic means, rather than drugs and medicines. Many graduates of *Hygienic* Colleges served as doctors in the Civil War and helped their patients recover more quickly by their hygienic methods.

The American Natural Hygiene Society now carries on the educational work of the movement through distribution of books published by its press and other publishers, pamphlets, annual public conventions and seminars and a chapter structure which functions in many large cities through the membership, dispensing *Natural Hygiene* education to the local people. Future goals of the Society are the establishment of colleges to train practitioners in the Hygienic System of health maintenance, institutes to care for the sick the hygienic way, and community centers for family living on an educational, social and recreational basis along *Natural Hygienic* lines.

THE DRUGLESS WAY TO BETTER HEALTH BOOKS
NATURAL HYGIENE PRESS PUBLICATIONS

A—FASTING CAN SAVE YOUR LIFE $1.75
H. M. Shelton. 191 pages. Part I: The basics and benefits of fasting. Tells how, when and where to fast for health restoration and weight reduction. Nine basic steps to a successful fast. Part II: Recovery through fasting from acute or chronic diseases such as asthma, arthritis, ulcers, migraine, high blood pressure, colitis, etc. An excellent introductory book on fasting.

B—YOU DON'T HAVE TO BE SICK! $1.45
J. D. Trop. 231 pages. A step-by-step routine for putting a healthful living program into action. Sample menus and party foods. A primer of Natural Hygiene.

C—HEALTH FOR THE MILLIONS $1.45
H. M. Shelton. 321 pages. 41 chapters on how the body functions, what it needs and what is harmful.

D—HYGIENIC CARE OF CHILDREN $1.95
H. M. Shelton. Over 400 pages. Paperback edition of a hardcover book long out of print. This is the parent's comprehensive guide to the rearing of healthy children and healthy pregnancy. Discusses harmful effects of inoculations.

E—EXERCISE! $1.95
H. M. Shelton. Paperback. A rare, comprehensive book on three levels: the history and role of formal exercise in maintaining good body functioning; how exercise aids in existing impairments by correcting weakened structural faults and muscles; profuse illustrations show how exercises are done. Reprinted from Volume 4 of The Hygienic System.

F—THE GREATEST HEALTH DISCOVERY $1.75
Natural Hygiene and its Evolution, Past, Present and Future. From the works of Sylvester Graham, Dr. R. T. Trall, H. M. Shelton and others, 241 pages, paperback. The health care revolution which started in 19th century America and solved the problem of disease and premature death. Contains portraits of the pioneers who were mostly medical doctors; 18 picture pages of the Hygienic way of life through the medium of traditional ANHS Convention; presents a practical plan for bringing unlimited health on a community level.

G—DICTIONARY OF MAN'S FOODS $2.25
William L. Esser. 179 pages, paperback. Descriptive alphabetic guide to fruits and vegetables and how to combine each for good digestion; table of food composition and nutritional values; seed sprouting instructions; food combining chart; list of food classifications; suggested menus for every day of the week. Separate chapters of fruits, vegetables, nuts, conservative cooking, the kitchen on a budget, best storing methods. Special color section shows varieties of breakfasts, lunches and dinners.

H—TOXEMIA: THE BASIC CAUSE OF ALL DISEASE $1.50
John H. Tilden. Reprinted 1974, 125 pages, paperback. An eminent medical doctor and Natural Hygiene pioneer tells how to get well and stay well the drugless way.

I—PROGRAM FOR DYNAMIC HEALTH $1.00
Compiled by T. C. Fry. A New York businessman gives his testimonial and tells how to practice Natural Hygiene.

J—FASTING FOR RENEWAL OF LIFE $2.25
H. M. Shelton. 320 pages, paperback. (1974) In depth details about what happens while the body is fasting and how this remarkable process, used since Biblical times, brings about renewal and healing.

K—DON'T GET STUCK $2.00
Hannah Allen. 110 pages. Legal and practical ways to avoid vaccinations, inoculations and injections in school and while traveling; plus germ theory refutation.

L—SUPERIOR FOODS, DIET PRINCIPLES, AND PRACTICES FOR PERFECT HEALTH $1.50

T. C. Fry. 64 pages. Reveals proper diets for maximum nutrition and good health, plus other points on efficient digestion.

M—THE HAPPY TRUTH ABOUT PROTEIN $1.00

Hannah Allen. 32 pages. Useful reference book charting amino acids and protein content of common foods; also details, varieties and quantities needed for optimal nutrition.

N—DIAGNOSIS: CANCER $1.00

Hannah Allen. 23 pages. Futility of surgery; hoax of cancer research; prevention through removal of cause.

O—PLEASE DON'T SMOKE IN OUR HOUSE $1.50

J. D. Trop. 128 pages. Undesirable physiological and social effects of the indulgence in the unnatural habit of smoking. Recommends ideal way to quit.

—HOMEMAKER'S GUIDE TO FOODS FOR PLEASURE AND HEALTH $2.50

Hannah Allen. 275 pages. Encyclopedic book about natural foods and Natural Hygiene. Menus, combinations, recipes, etc.

OTHER NATURAL HYGIENE PUBLICATIONS

Q—FOOD COMBINING MADE EASY $1.50

H. M. Shelton. 71 pages. Everything you need to know to avoid the after-meal discomfort of heartburn, bloating, flatulence, acid indigestion, etc., with proper food combining.

R—SUPERIOR NUTRITION $3.25

H. M. Shelton. 197 pages. Condensed version of Volume 2 of The Hygienic System. Includes basic nutritional needs of the body, processed versus natural foods, organic versus inorganic; requirements of starches, proteins, vitamins, minerals, amino acids; proper diet for well-being, fasting, feeding babies naturally, avoiding gluttony, how to plan and eat meals, menus, feeding the sick.

T—FIT FOOD FOR MAN $.50

Arthur Andrews. 16 pages. Explains why man functions best on a fruit, nut and vegetable diet. Anatomical comparison chart shows how differences in various animal species (including human beings) determine what type of food they are constituted to eat; shows the carnivora, omnivora, herbivora, and frugivora (man).

—MEDICAL DRUGS ON TRIAL? VERDICT "GUILTY" $2.25

Keki R. Sidhwa. 256 pages. An expose of the present day practice of medicine; the drug industry; and food technology.

JA—THE HYGIENIC SYSTEM: VOLUME I $5.00

H. M. Shelton, 352 pages. (Reprint, revised 1972) The laws governing human life; care of the organs of the body; introduction gives brief historical background of the Hygienic Movement.

JB—SYPHILIS: THE WEREWOLF OF MEDICINE $4.50

H. M. Shelton. 150 pages, Gives the true cause of syphilis and shows why disease or cure is a myth. The cure is deadlier than the disease.

C—LIVING LIFE TO LIVE IT LONGER $3.00

H. M. Shelton. 139 pages. How to live more joyfully and with fulfillment via Natural Hygiene.

D—FASTING FOR HEALTH AND LONG LIFE $3.00

H. M. Carrington. 151 pages. Facts about fasting in abbreviated form; covers fasting pros and cons, recovery of colds and other ailments; many diets reviewed; effects of fasting on the body, fasting crises, breaking the fast, etc.

JE—AN INTRODUCTION TO NATURAL HYGIENE $2.00

H. M. Shelton. 92 pages. Basic reading for understanding the principles underlying the Natural Hygiene system of health maintenance and recovery; defines health and disease, reveals the healing powers of the body, methods of care, feeding and fasting.

JF—THERAPEUTIC FASTING $2.50

Arnold De Vries. 77 pages. A scientific survey of the value of fasting from the writings of 39 different authors. Statistics are given on the effects of fasting for a host of diseases, as gleaned from Natural Hygiene doctors. Each disease lists the number of cases involved in the study, the number of cases which improved or were remedied, and the number of cases which were not helped.

XA—THE HYGIENIC SYSTEM: VOLUME II (FOOD AND FEEDING) $7.50

H. M. Shelton. 591 pages. A complete guide to correct use of natural foods and feeding from infancy on. Starts with food elements, vitamins, calories, minerals, organic foods, proteins, starches, etc.; covers proper food combining for maximum digestion; raw versus cooked foods; menus; infant feeding; etc. Promises a startling awakening for the reader interested in human nutrition.

XC—NATURAL HYGIENE: MAN'S PRISTINE WAY OF LIFE $7.50

H. M. Shelton. 638 pages. A complete book on the requirements of the body for health maintenance and recovery. Includes historical background of the Hygienic Movement.

XD—HUMAN BEAUTY: ITS CULTURE AND HYGIENE $12.50

H. M. Shelton. 1039 pages. The important relationship between good body functioning and genetic beauty. Over 100 illustrations. Discusses care of the body and gives exercises for neck, shoulders, arms, chest, back muscles, etc.

XF—CORRECT FOOD COMBINING PLACE MAT (45¢ P&H) $1.50

12 x 18 plastic coated. Foods shown in color, indicating good, fair and poor combinations for efficient digestion. Side Two explains combinations and classifies proteins, carbohydrates, starches, fats, etc. with other useful food information.

XH—A GIFT OF LOVE $7.50

J. D. Trop. 320 pages, hardcover. A documented story of 86 Australian World War II orphans who were raised naturally as an experiment and who subsequently set many health records. A True Gift of Love to humanity by L. O. Bailey and Madge Cockburn—pictures.

DR. SHELTON'S HYGIENIC REVIEW

$7.50/Yr. ($8.00/Yr. Canada, Foreign)

A monthly magazine edited and published by H. M. Shelton. Vital articles on the cause of diseases, how to maintain health, errors of medical practices.

● ADD 25¢ TO EACH BOOK FOR POSTAGE AND HANDLING CHARGES. Write for special discounts on quantity lots.

● When writing for information of a general nature, please include a stamped, self-addressed envelope and 25¢ to help defray cost of postage and handling. All prices subject to change. Allow 3 to 4 weeks for delivery (overseas up to 90 days).

NATURAL HYGIENE PRESS
BOOK ORDER FORM U

☐	A—FASTING CAN SAVE YOUR LIFE	$1.75
☐	B—YOU DON'T HAVE TO BE SICK!	$1.45
☐	C—HEALTH FOR THE MILLIONS	$1.45
☐	D—HYGIENIC CARE OF CHILDREN	$1.95
☐	E—EXERCISE!	$1.95
☐	F—THE GREATEST HEALTH DISCOVERY	$1.75
☐	G—DICTIONARY OF MAN'S FOOD	$2.25
☐	H—TOXEMIA	$1.50
☐	I—PROGRAM FOR DYNAMIC HEALTH	$1.00
☐	J—FASTING FOR RENEWAL OF LIFE	$2.25
☐	K—DON'T GET STUCK—VIA VACCINATIONS AND INJECTIONS	$2.00
☐	L—SUPERIOR FOODS, DIET PRINCIPLES AND PRACTICES, ETC.	$1.50
☐	M—THE HAPPY TRUTH ABOUT PROTEIN	$1.00
☐	N—DIAGNOSIS CANCER—ESCAPE FEAR VIA NATURAL HYGIENE	$1.00
☐	O—PLEASE DON'T SMOKE IN OUR HOUSE	$1.50
☐	P—FOODS FOR PLEASURE & HEALTH; HANDBOOK FOR HYGIENIC LIVING	$2.50
☐	Q—FOOD COMBINING MADE EASY	$1.50
☐	R—SUPERIOR NUTRITION	$3.25
☐	T—FIT FOOD FOR MAN	.50
☐	U—MEDICAL DRUGS ON TRIAL	$2.25
☐	JA—THE HYGIENIC SYSTEM, VOL. I	$5.00
☐	JB—SYPHILIS: THE WEREWOLF OF MEDICINE	$4.50
☐	JC—LIVING LIFE TO LIVE IT LONGER	$3.00
☐	JD—FASTING FOR HEALTH AND LONG LIFE	$3.00
☐	JE—AN INTRODUCTION TO NATURAL HYGIENE	$2.00
☐	JF—THERAPEUTIC FASTING	$2.50
☐	XA—THE HYGIENIC SYSTEM, VOL. II—COMPLETE GUIDE TO FOOD AND FEEDING	$7.50
☐	XC—NATURAL HYGIENE: MAN'S PRISTINE WAY OF LIFE	$7.50
☐	XD—HUMAN BEAUTY: ITS CULTURE AND HYGIENE	$12.50
☐	XF—CORRECT FOOD COMBINING PLACE MAT (PLUS 45¢ P&H)	$1.50
☐	XH—A GIFT OF LOVE	$7.50
☐	DR. SHELTON'S HYGIENIC REVIEW ($8/YR. Canada, Foreign)	$7.50/YR.

● ADD 25¢ TO EACH BOOK FOR POSTAGE AND HANDLING CHARGES.

● SEE NEXT PAGE FOR ORDER BLANK

TOTAL $_____

NOTICE TO THE READER

If after reading this book, you feel the vital knowledge which it contains deserves to be made widely known, you are urged to become a member of the American Natural Hygiene Society and help to contribute to this worthy cause for the benefit of mankind. (Contributions, wills, bequests are tax exempt.)

As a membership bonus we will send this book or any other N.H.P. publication in value up to $1.95 to anyone of your choice. Fill out the application below and mail your remittance of $11.00 for your membership and the bonus book. Outside U.S.A.—$12.00.

☐—Please enroll me as a member of your worthy cause. Enclosed find $11.00 *payable in U. S. $ to A.N.H.S.* for the annual *membership and bonus book.*

☐—BOOK ORDER—Enclosed find $_____ for books indicated on order form "U" Payable in U. S. $ to NATURAL HYGIENE PRESS.

Name_____
(please print)

Address_____

City, State, Zip_____

Phone No._____Age_____

SEND BONUS BOOK TITLED_____

_____

To_____
(please print)

Address_____

City, State, Zip_____

AMERICAN NATURAL HYGIENE SOCIETY, Dept U.
1920 IRVING PARK ROAD, CHICAGO, ILL. 60613

U